Clinical Care Record Book For Midwifery Program

(In accordance with INC Guidelines)

Priscilla John MSc (OBG)
Lecturer
Pal College of Nursing and Medical Sciences Haldwani
Nainital, Uttarakhand, India

Rekha Kumari MSc (OBG)
Lecturer
Pal College of Nursing and Medical Sciences Haldwani
Nainital, Uttarakhand, India

With Guidance of: **Dr Ratna Prakash** PhD PGDHE
Principal
Pal College of Nursing and Medical Sciences Haldwani
Nainital, Uttarakhand, India

Foreword
Ashok Pal

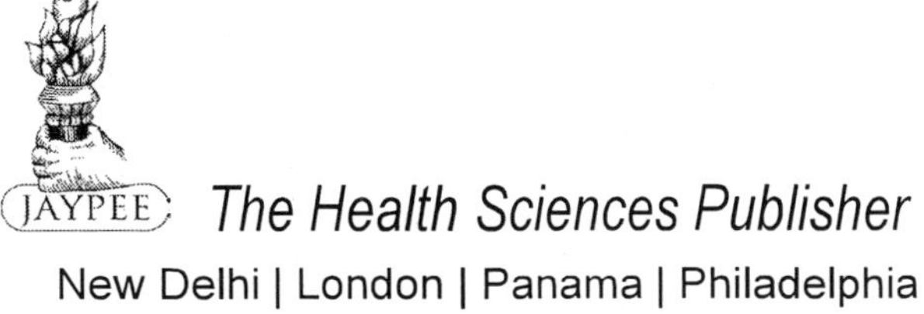

New Delhi | London | Panama | Philadelphia

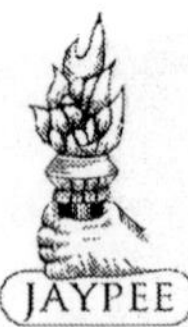

Jaypee Brothers Medical Publishers (P) Ltd

Headquarters

Jaypee Brothers Medical Publishers (P) Ltd
4838/24, Ansari Road, Daryaganj
New Delhi 110 002, India
Phone: +91-11-43574357
Fax: +91-11-43574314
Email: jaypee@jaypeebrothers.com

Overseas Offices

J.P. Medical Ltd
83, Victoria Street, London
SW1H 0HW (UK)
Phone: +44-20 3170 8910
Fax: +44-(0)20 3008 6180
Email: info@jpmedpub.com

Jaypee-Highlights Medical Publishers Inc
City of Knowledge, Bld. 237, Clayton
Panama City, Panama
Phone: +1 507-301-0496
Fax: +1 507-301-0499
Email: cservice@jphmedical.com

Jaypee Medical Inc
The Bourse
111, South Independence Mall East
Suite 835, Philadelphia, PA 19106, USA
Phone: +1 267-519-9789
Email: joe.rusko@jaypeebrothers.com

Jaypee Brothers Medical Publishers (P) Ltd
17/1-B, Babar Road, Block-B, Shaymali
Mohammadpur, Dhaka-1207
Bangladesh
Mobile: +08801912003485
Email: jaypeedhaka@gmail.com

Jaypee Brothers Medical Publishers (P) Ltd
Bhotahity, Kathmandu, Nepal
Phone: +977-9741283608
Email: Kathmandu@jaypeebrothers.com

Website: www.jaypeebrothers.com
Website: www.jaypeedigital.com

Clinical Care Record Book for Midwifery Program (In accordance with INC Guidelines)

First Edition: **2015, Reprint 2024**

ISBN : 978-93-5152-800-5

Printed in India

Foreword

Clinical Record Book is the compilation prepared for GNM and BSc Nursing Students. These students, on completion of the course, would support the health care delivery system at all health care arenas, where mother and child health is a major concern. GNM and BSc Nursing Professionals function as significant members of the Health Team at these levels. Hence, it is important to prepare the students of these courses suitably for performing their roles in the team.

The chapters are well thought of preliminaries to gently guide student's clinical learning experiences from 'known to unknown and simple to complex' phenomena that take place during birthing process. The language used is student friendly, materials are organized in logical sequence and learning experiences are designed to incorporate all the aspects of mother and child care from the conception to child birth and extending to new born care.

A well developed documentation system serves many purposes. Systematic documentation of learning experiences is an essential skill for all professional disciplines. The written documents are used as tools for evaluating student's learning. This compilation fulfils all these purposes, as aimed for.

It is a commendable task. I congratulate Mrs Priscilla John and Miss Rekha Kumari, teaching faculty of Pal College of Nursing and Medical Sciences for their thoughtful and organized efforts for facilitating student's learning.

Ashok Pal BE (Civil Engineering)
Director
Pal College of Nursing and Medical Sciences Haldwani
Nainital, Uttarakhand, India

Preface

This Clinical Record Book is prepared to accomplish the needs of all Midwifery students in their learning experiences. The content is arranged keeping in mind INC syllabus, requirements of GNM and BSc Nursing course and Indian Nursing Council standards.

This compilation aims to direct student's clinical reasoning in logical sequence with brief review of structural description of the body parts of mother and baby, participating in the process of birth. Thus, the initial chapters present brief review notes on the essential elements of birthing process, viz. female pelvis; fetal skull; fetal circulation and fetal lie. Following the chapters are organized incorporating the improvised steps of nursing process.

A brief description of the record book contents:

The logbook is designed to help undergraduate students to provide safe, sensitive and thoughtful care to their mother and child client unit.

The teaching and clinical supervision of teachers and efficient curriculum management enable the student to meet the unique requirement for practical and clinical aspects of midwifery.

Midwife is the person who assists women in childbirth. The students of this course must be capable and skillful in providing quality health care services.

Our main concern while compiling this clinical care record book is to consider the requirement of a midwifery students, their development of knowledge and skill in caring for each and every woman in pregnancy, labour and postpartum period. We hope that the minimum essential information added in this complication would benefit GNM and BSc nursing students as a record of their practical work.

I hope the content of this book will support the midwifery students in providing compassionate care to woman in pregnancy and newborn. I request all viewers and students to provide me with comments about each chapter, so that necessary changes could be done in next edition.

Dr Ratna Prakash

Acknowledgments

'We express our gratitude to Almighty God. For His grace and blessings, who has been the guiding force behind all our efforts'.

Our heartfelt thanks to Dr Ratna Prakash Professor, Principal of Pal College of Nursing and Medical Sciences for the encouragement, inspirations and support for taking up this project and guiding till its completion.

We express our Sincere Gratitude to Mr Ashok Pal, Director of the Institute for his constant encouragement in this work and for accepting to write the foreword for this book.

We are indebted to our colleagues for enriching this work by their expert suggestions and generally being there for us whenever we needed to fall back for their support.

We have put forth our sincere effort in compiling materials for *Clinical Care Record Book for Midwifery Program*, for the benefit of our students. We acknowledge and appreciate their indirect contribution in refining the materials as we got insights from their difficulty in using the formats.

PAL COLLEGE OF NURSING & MEDICAL SCIENCES
HALDWANI, NAINITAL

Clinical Care Record Book for Midwifery Program

(In accordance with INC Guidelines)

Name of the Student ....

....

....

Name of the Course ....

Year ....

Roll No. ....

....

Internal Examiner

....

External Examiner

PAL COLLEGE OF NURSING & MEDICAL SCIENCES
HALDWANI, NAINITAL

Requirement for Midwifery Student

Casebook of Obstetrics and Gynaecological

Female Pelvis

Fetal Skull

Fetal Circulation

Lie

Antenatal Assessment

Normal Delivery Witnessed

Abnormal Delivery Witnessed

Vaginal Examination

Episiotomies and Skin Suturing

Caesarean Section Witnessed

Insertion of IUD/Cu-T

Care Studies

1. Antenatal Care Study	30
2. Conducted Care Study	20
3. Postnatal and Neonatal Care Study	20

Signature of Internal Examiner

Signature of External Examiner

Signature of Principal

Contents

FEMALE PELVIS

FEMALE PELVIS

The pelvic girdle, a basin shape cavity, is a bony ring between the movable vertebrae of the vertebral column which is supports, and the lower limbs that it rest on. It contains and protects the bladder, rectum and internal reproductive organ.

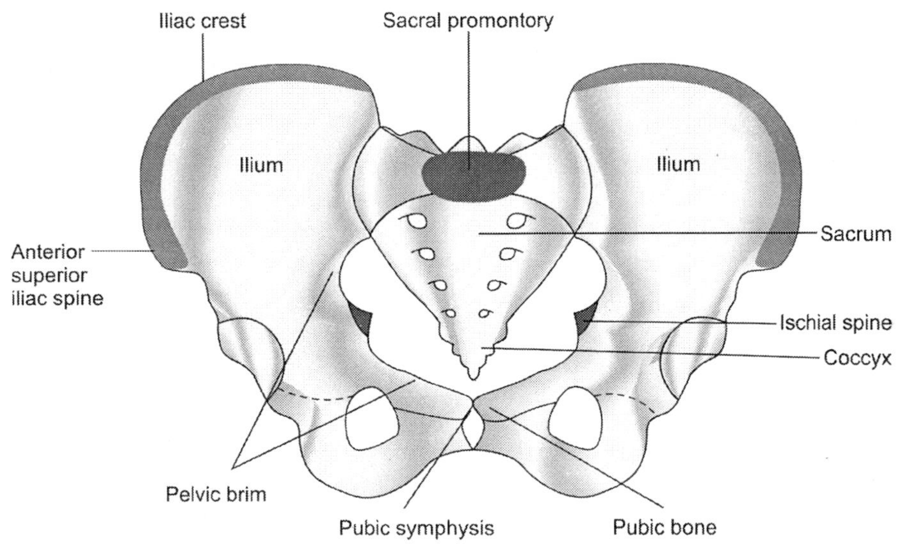

Fig. 1.1: Female pelvis

PELVIC BONES

Total Four Bones:

1. Two innominated bones
2. One sacrum
3. One coccyx

1. Innominate bone is made-up of three bones

a. Ilium
b. Iischium
c. Pubic bone

a. Ilium: It is the large flared out part. It is formed by:

(i) Iliac crest
(ii) Anterior superior iliac spine
(iii) Anterior inferior iliac spine
(iv) Posterior superior iliac spine
(v) Posterior inferior iliac spine
(vi) Iliac fossa

b. Ischium is the thick lower part

(i) Ischial tuberosity
(ii) Ischila spines
(iii) Superior ramus
(iv) Inferior ramus
(v) Symphysis pubis
(vi) Pubic arch
(vii) Obturator foramen

c. **Pubic bone: Two pubic bone joints and form Symphysis pubis**
   (i) Acetabulum
   (ii) Superior ramus
   (iii) Greater sciatic notches
   (iv) Lesser sciatic notches

2. **Sacrum is a wedge-shaped bone consisting of five fused vertebrae**
   a. Sacral promontory
   b. Sacral ala or wing
   c. Hollow of sacrum
   d. Sacral foramina
   e. Four pairs of holes or foramina

3. **Coccyx is a vestigial tail:** It consists of four fused vertebrae, forming a small triangular bone.

PELVIC JOINTS

1. One symphysis pubis
2. Two sacroiliac joint
3. One sacrococcygeal joint

PELVIC LIGAMENT

1. Interpubic ligament
2. Sacro-coccygeal ligament
3. Sacroiliac ligament
4. Sacrotuberous ligament
5. Sacrospinous ligament

REGIONS OF PELVIC

It is divided into two parts

1. True pelvis
2. False pelvis

1. **True Pelvis:** It is the bony canal through which the fetus must pass during birth.
   a. Inlet or pelvic brim
   b. Pelvic cavity
   c. Outlet

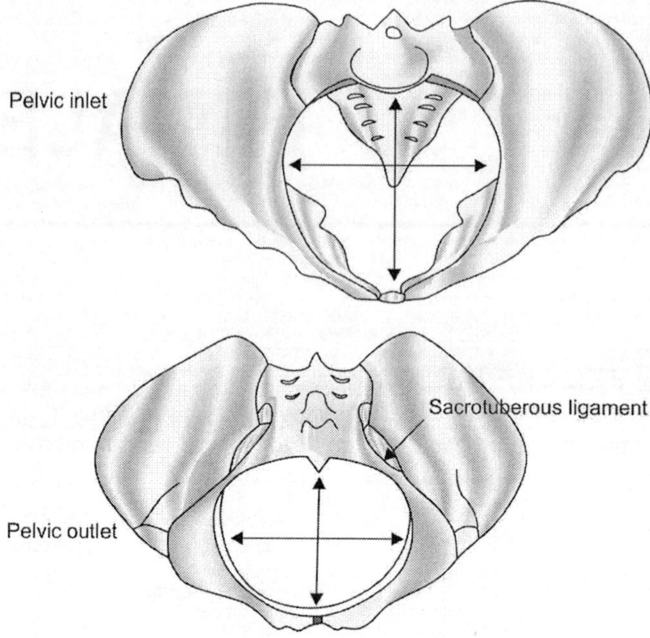

Fig. 1.2: True pelvis

a. **Pelvic brim:** The pelvic brim has fixed point called as landmark. Which commencing posteriorly these are:
   (i) Sacral promontory
   (ii) Sacral wing
   (iii) Sacroiliac joint
   (iv) Iliopectineal line
   (v) Iliopectineal eminence
   (vi) Superior ramus of pubis
   (vii) Pubic tubercal
   (viii) Symphysis pubis

b. **Pelvic cavity**
   (i) Symphysis pubis
   (ii) Curve of ligament
   (iii) Ligament and soft tissues

c. **Pelvic outlet**
   (i) Anatomical outlet
   (ii) Obstetrical outlet

PELVIC DIAMETERS

Regions	Brim	Cavity	Outlet
Anteroposterior diameter	11 cm	12 cm	13 cm
Oblique diameter	12 cm	12 cm	12 cm
Transverse diameter	13 cm	12 cm	11 cm

TYPES OF PELVIS

1. Gynaecoid pelvis
2. Android pelvis
3. Platypelloid pelvis
4. Anthropoid pelvis

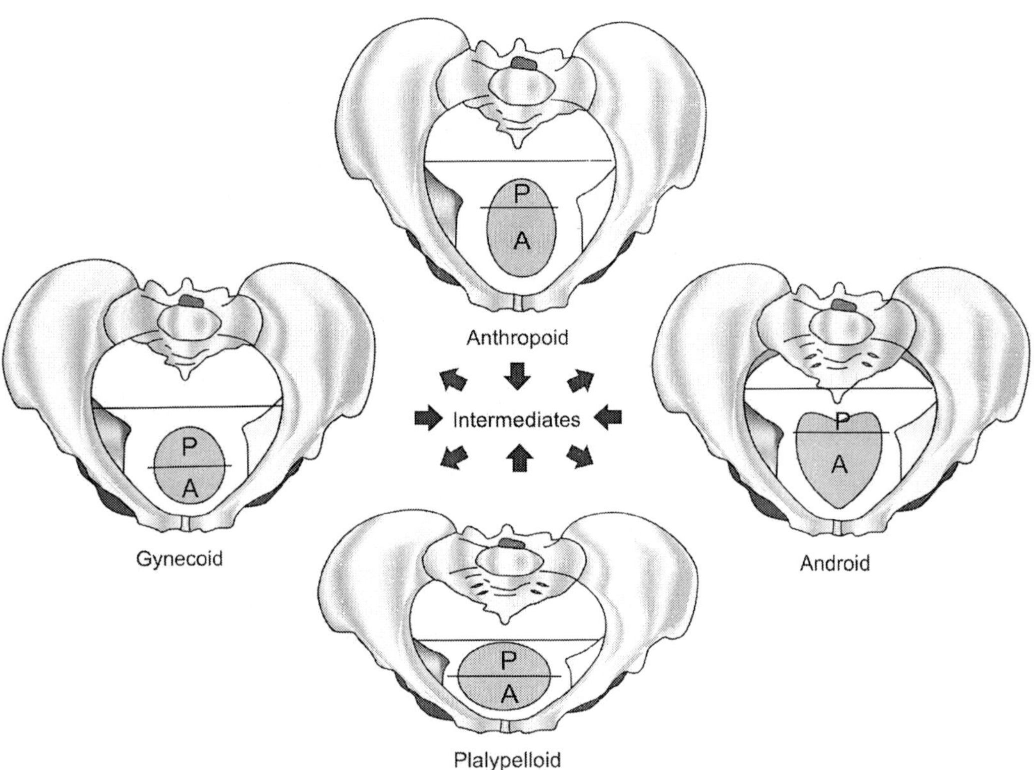

Fig. 1.3: Types of pelvis

FETAL SKULL

The fetal head is large in relation to the fetal body compared with the adult. The fetal skull contains the delicate brain, which may be subjected to great pressure as the head pass through the birth canal.

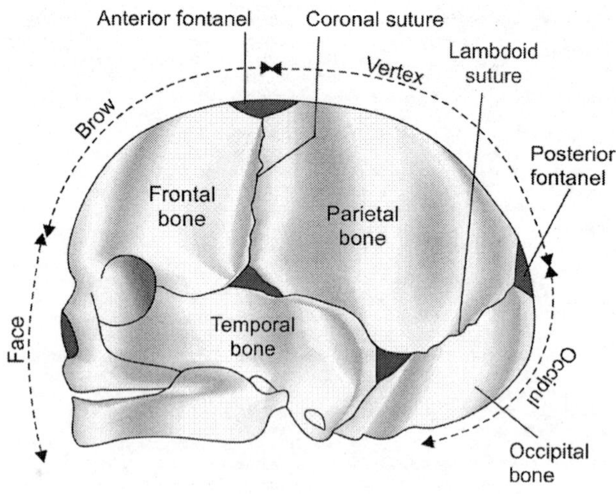

Fig. 2.1: Fetal skull

BONES OF THE VAULT

1. Two frontal bones
2. Two parietal bones
3. One occipital bone
4. Two temporal bones

SUTURES

These are formed when two bones joint together:

1. Frontal suture
2. Sagittal suture
3. Coronal suture
4. Lambdoidal suture

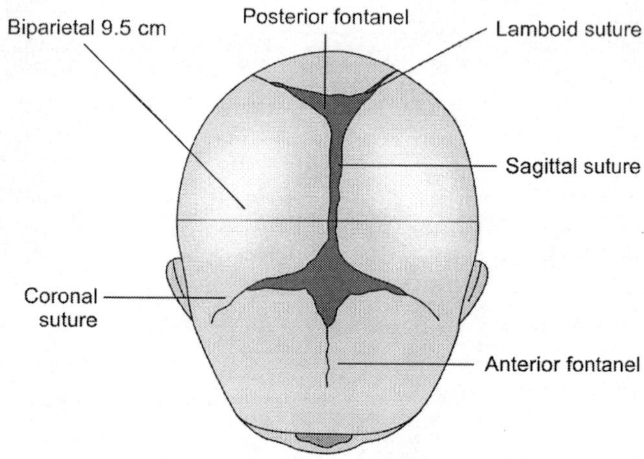

Fig. 2.2: Sutures and fontanelles

FONTANELLES

These are formed when two or more suture joins together.

1. Anterior fontanelle
2. Posterior fontanelle

DIAMETERS OF FETAL SKULL

It is divided into two parts:

1. Anteroposterior Diameter (Total Six Diameter)
2. Transverse Diameter (Total Two Diameter)

Diameters	Length (cm)
• **Anteroposterior diameter**	
– SOB: Suboccipitobregmatic	09.5
– DOF: Suboccipitofrontal	10.5
– OF: Occipitofrontal	11.0
– MV: Mentovertical	13.5
– SMV: Submentovertical	11.5
– SMB: Submentobregmatic	9.5

- **Transverse diameter**
  - Biparietal Diameter 9.5
  - Bitemporal Diameter 8.2

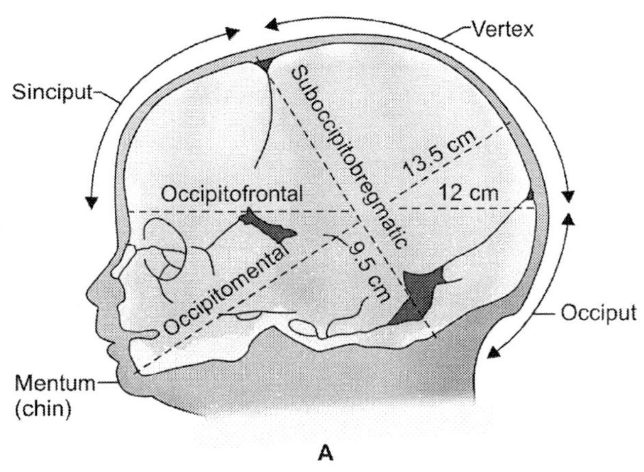

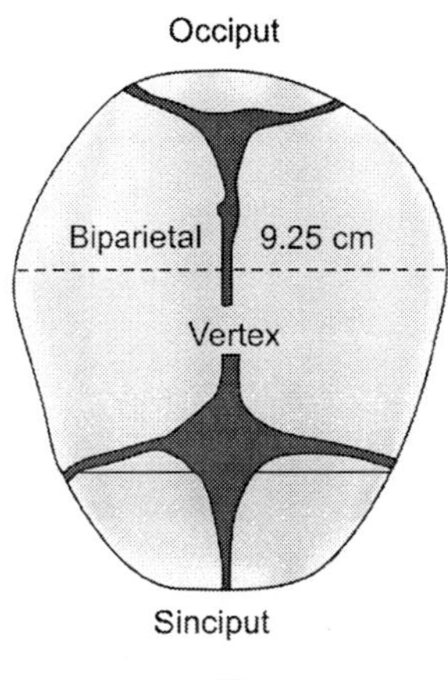

Figs 2.3A and B: (A) Anteroposterior diameter (B) Transverse diameter

FETAL CIRCULATION

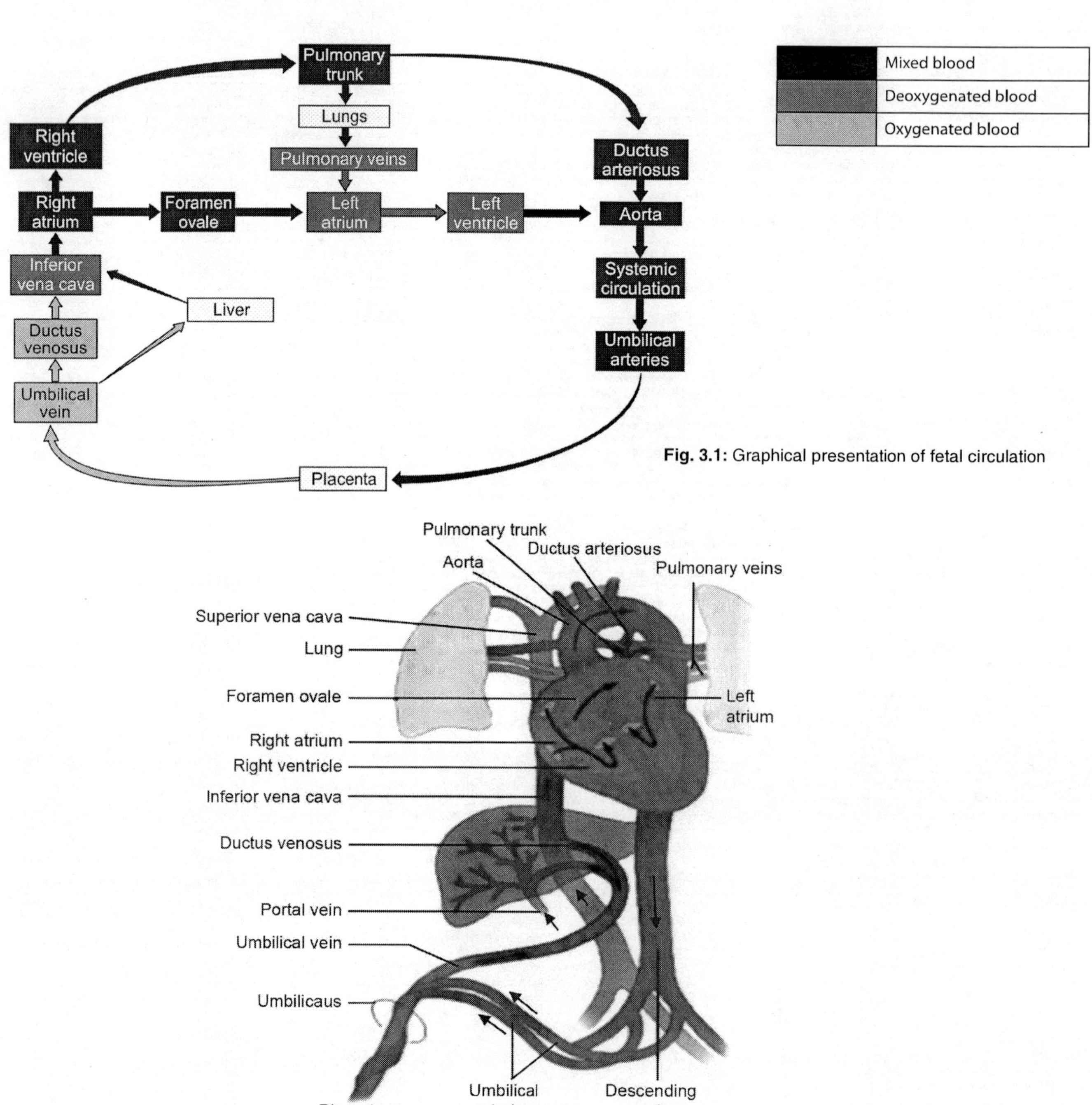

Fig. 3.1: Graphical presentation of fetal circulation

3.2: Fetal circulation

LIE

The lie of the fetus is the relationship between the long axis of the fetus and the long axis of the uterus. In the majority of cases the lie is longitudinal owing to the ovoid shape of the uterus, the remainder are oblique or transverse. Oblique lie, when the fetus lies diagonally across the long axis of the uterus. When the lie is transverse the fetus lies at right angles across the long axis of the uterus. These lie is divided in three parts.

1. **Longitudinal Lie**
   a. Breech
   b. Vertex
2. **Transverse Lie**
3. **Oblique Lie**

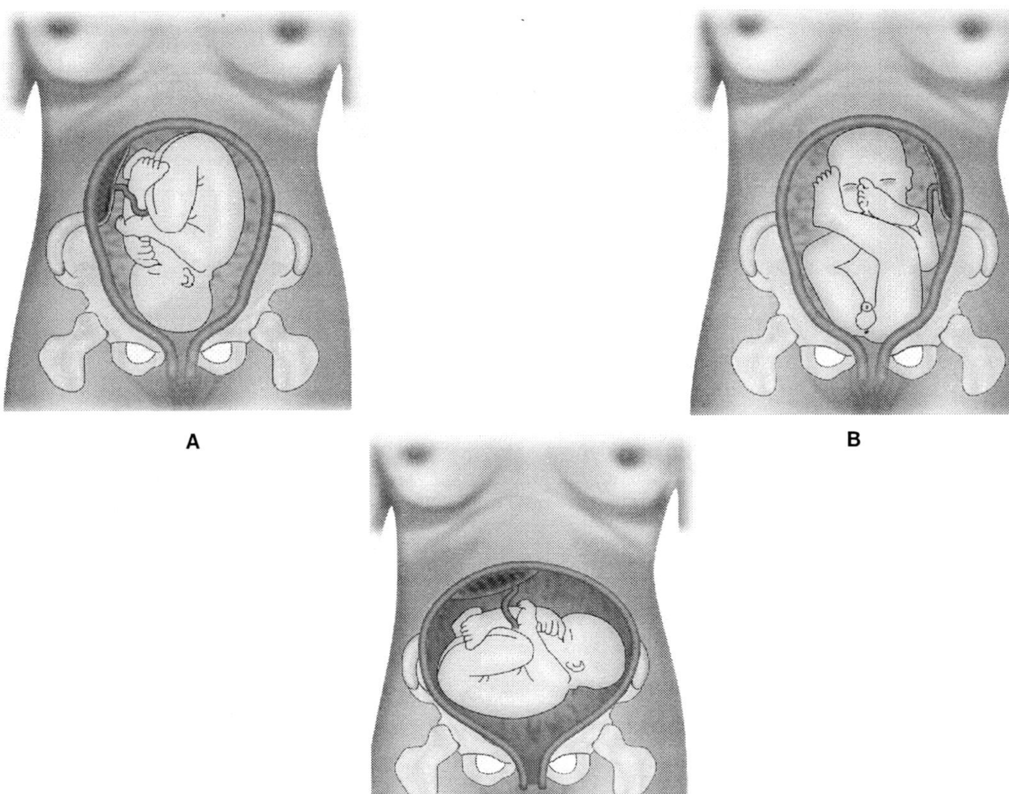

Figs 3.3A to C: (A) Longitudinal lie: Vertex presentation (B) Longitudinal lie: Breech presentation (C) Transverse lie: Shoulder presentation

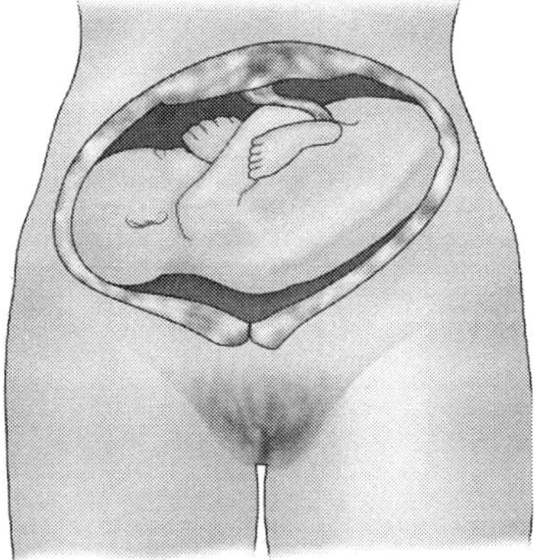

Fig. 3.4: Transverse lie

ANTENATAL ASSESSMENT

S. No.	Date	Reg.No.	Name of the Mother	Age	GPLA	BP	Urine		Weight group	Blood			Gestational Age (weeks)	Ht.of Fundus in cms	Presentation	Position	Engagement	FHS/ min	Treatment	Sign of Teacher
							Albumin	Sugar		Hb	Group	VDRL								

Contd...

Contd...

S. No.	Date	Reg.No.	Name of the Mother	Age	GPLA	BP	Urine		Weight group	Blood			Gestational Age (weeks)	Ht.of Fundus in cms	Presentation	Position	Engagement	FHS/min	Treatment	Sign of Teacher
							Albumin	Sugar		Hb	Group	VDRL								

NORMAL DELIVERY WITNESSED

S. No.	Date	Reg. No.	Name of the Mother	Age	GPLA	Presentation	Position	Time of Delivery	Gen-der	Weight of Baby	Type of Delivery	Conducted By	Sign of Teacher

ABNORMAL DELIVERY WITNESSED

S. No.	Date	Reg. No	Information related to Mother								Information related to the Newborn			Special Note	Teacher's Signature
			Name of the Mother	Age (Yrs)	GPLA	Foetal Position	Foetal Presenta-tion	Time of Delivery	Type of Delivery	Conducted By	Gender	Weight (kg)	APGAR Score		

VAGINAL EXAMINATIONS

S. No.	Date	Reg. No	Name of the Mother	Age	GPLA	Cervix		Membranes	Presentation	Station of Presentation Part	Position of Occiput	Sign of Teacher
						Effacement	Dilation					

EPISIOTOMY AND SKIN SUTURING

S.No.	Date	Reg. No	Name of the Mother	Age	GPLA	Type of Delivery	Sutured With	No. of Suture	Signature of Teacher

CAESAREAN SECTION WITNESSED

S. No.	Date	Reg.No	Name of the Mother	Age	GPLA	Presentation	Position	Time of Delivery	Gender of Baby	Wgt. of Baby	Operation Notes and Indication	Condition of Mother	Condition of Baby	Conducted By	Sign of Teacher

INSERTION OF INTRAUTERINE DEVICE

S. No.	Date	Reg. No	Name of the Mother	Age	GPLA	Type of IUD	Life Span of IUD	Date of Removal of IUD	Health Education	Remarks	Signature of Teacher

CU-T INSERTION CASE NO.

IDENTIFICATION DATA

Hospital: ....
Name of the Client/Mother: ....
W/O: ....
Reg No: ....
Age: ....
Religion: ....
Address: ....
Time of Cu-T Insertion after: Child Birth/Abortion/MTP/D&E ....
GPLA: ....
Age of the Last Child Born: ....

PRELIMINARIES FOR CU-T INSERTION

- Consent taken for the Contraceptive Choice: Yes/No ....
- Evacuation of Bladder:-done/Not done. ....
- History of Medical Surgical: ....
- Vaginal Examination: ....
  a. Shape of Uterus. ....
  b. Position of the Uterus ....
  c. Size of the Uterus ....
  d. Condition of Cervix ....
  e. Signs of Infection ....
- Consent taken for the Contraceptive Choice: Yes/No. ....
- Evacuation of Bladder: Done/Not Done ....

STEPS OF CU-T INSERTION:

....
....

ADVICES TO THE MOTHER:

....
....

TIME OF CU-T REMOVAL:

....
....

FOLLOW-UP:

....
....

Teacher's Signature ....

CU-T INSERTION CASE NO.

IDENTIFICATION DATA

Hospital: ....

Name of the Client/Mother: ....

W/O: ....

Reg No: ....

Age: ....

Religion: ....

Address: ....

Time of Cu-T Insertion after: Child Birth/Abortion/MTP/D&E ....

GPLA: ....

Age of the Last Child Born: ....

PRELIMINARIES FOR CU-T INSERTION

- Consent taken for the Contraceptive Choice: Yes/No ....
- Evacuation of Bladder:-done/Not done. ....
- History of Medical Surgical: ....
- Vaginal Examination: ....
  a. Shape of Uterus. ....
  b. Position of the Uterus ....
  c. Size of the Uterus ....
  d. Condition of Cervix ....
  e. Signs of Infection ....
- Consent taken for the Contraceptive Choice: Yes/No. ....
- Evacuation of Bladder: Done/Not Done ....

STEPS OF CU-T INSERTION:

....

....

ADVICES TO THE MOTHER:

....

....

TIME OF CU-T REMOVAL:

....

....

FOLLOW-UP:

....

....

Teacher's Signature ....

CU-T INSERTION CASE NO.

IDENTIFICATION DATA

Hospital: ....
Name of the Client/Mother: ....
W/O: ....
Reg No: ....
Age: ....
Religion: ....
Address: ....
Time of Cu-T Insertion after: Child Birth/Abortion/MTP/D&E...
GPLA: ....
Age of the Last Child Born: ....

PRELIMINARIES FOR CU-T INSERTION

- Consent taken for the Contraceptive Choice: Yes/No ....
- Evacuation of Bladder:-done/Not done. ....
- History of Medical Surgical: ....
- Vaginal Examination: ....
    a. Shape of Uterus. ....
    b. Position of the Uterus ....
    c. Size of the Uterus ....
    d. Condition of Cervix ....
    e. Signs of Infection ....
- Consent taken for the Contraceptive Choice: Yes/No. ....
- Evacuation of Bladder: Done/Not Done ....

STEPS OF CU-T INSERTION:

....

....

ADVICES TO THE MOTHER:

....

....

TIME OF CU-T REMOVAL:

....

....

FOLLOW-UP:

....

....

Teacher's Signature...

CU-T INSERTION CASE NO.

IDENTIFICATION DATA

Hospital:..........

Name of the Client/Mother:..........

W/O:..........

Reg No:..........

Age:..........

Religion:..........

Address:..........

Time of Cu-T Insertion after: Child Birth/Abortion/MTP/D&E..........

GPLA:..........

Age of the Last Child Born:..........

PRELIMINARIES FOR CU-T INSERTION

- Consent taken for the Contraceptive Choice: Yes/No ....
- Evacuation of Bladder:-done/Not done. ....
- History of Medical Surgical:..........
- Vaginal Examination:..........
  a. Shape of Uterus. ....
  b. Position of the Uterus..........
  c. Size of the Uterus..........
  d. Condition of Cervix..........
  e. Signs of Infection ....
- Consent taken for the Contraceptive Choice: Yes/No. ....
- Evacuation of Bladder: Done/Not Done..........

STEPS OF CU-T INSERTION:

....

....

ADVICES TO THE MOTHER:

....

....

TIME OF CU-T REMOVAL:

....

....

FOLLOW-UP:

....

....

Teacher's Signature..........

CU-T INSERTION CASE NO.

IDENTIFICATION DATA

Hospital: ....

Name of the Client/Mother: ....

W/O: ....

Reg No: ....

Age: ....

Religion: ....

Address: ....

Time of Cu-T Insertion after: Child Birth/Abortion/MTP/D&E ....

GPLA: ....

Age of the Last Child Born: ....

PRELIMINARIES FOR CU-T INSERTION

- Consent taken for the Contraceptive Choice: Yes/No ....
- Evacuation of Bladder:-done/Not done. ....
- History of Medical Surgical: ....
- Vaginal Examination: ....
  a. Shape of Uterus. ....
  b. Position of the Uterus ....
  c. Size of the Uterus ....
  d. Condition of Cervix ....
  e. Signs of Infection ....
- Consent taken for the Contraceptive Choice: Yes/No. ....
- Evacuation of Bladder: Done/Not Done ....

STEPS OF CU-T INSERTION:

....

....

ADVICES TO THE MOTHER:

....

....

TIME OF CU-T REMOVAL:

....

....

FOLLOW-UP:

....

....

Teacher's Signature ....

CARE STUDIES

- **Antenatal Care Study**
- **Conducted Care Study**
- **Postnatal and Neonatal Care Study**

ANTENATAL CARE STUDY

IDENTIFICATION DATA

Name of Mother...

Reg. No:..

Age: ....

Gravida: ....

Para:..

Diagnosis: ....

Date of Admission:...

Date of Discharge: ....

PAST MENSTRUAL HISTORY

LMP ....EDD ....Cycle...

HEALTH HISTORY

1. Past Obstetrical History..

   ....

   ....

2. Present Pregnancy History

   - I-trimester...

     ....

     ....

   - II-trimester..

     ....

     ....

- III-trimester...

....

....

3. Past Medical History ....

....

....

4. Present Surgical History. ....

....

....

5. Past Surgical History. ....

....

....

6. Family History. ....

....

....

7. Personal History. ....

....

....

OBSTETRICAL HISTORY

S.No.	Year	Abortion	Prem	F.T.	Type of Labour and Mode of Delivery	Gender	Live or Still Birth	Remark

ANTENATAL ATTENDANCES

LMP............................ EDD...Gestation at 1st visit.................. wk

Date	Wt	BP	FHS	Weeks	Fundal Height	Presentation	Treatments and Remarks

GENERAL EXAMINATION

Poor/Fair/Good

Height: .... cms Weight:............................Kgs

BP: mm Hg .... Temp: ....Pulse:..................... /Min Resp:........................./Min

Urine: Alb .... Sugar...

PHYSICAL EXAMINATION

HEAD: Hygiene...

Injury...

Surgery...

Infection ....

Any other ....

FACE: Expression...

Symmetry...

Chloasma ....

Scar...

EYES: Field of Vision...

Vision ....

Conjunctiva ....

Sclera. ....

Periorbital Oedema ....

Complaints if any ....

EARS: Hygiene..........

Hearing..........

Pain..........

Wax..........

Discharge..........

Surgery..........

Complaints if any..........

NOSE: Septal Deviation..........

Discharge..........

Bleeding..........

Polyp..........

Hygiene..........

Complaints if any..........

MOUTH: Lips: Colour.......... Texture..........

Stomatitis:..........

Hygiene:..........

Halitosis:..........

Tongue:..........

Teeth: Stain..........Symmetry.......... Caries..........Extractions..........

Pain ....Fillings. ....

GUMS: Colour..........

Bleeding..........

Gingivitis..........

Complaints if any..........

NECK: Hygiene..........

Nodes..........

Glands..........

Thyroid..........

Jugular Veins..........

Scar..........

Complaints if any..........

CHEST: Shape...

Scar. ....

LIMBS: Upper-Symmetry...

Tremors ....

Nails...

Hygiene...

Infection ....

Ulnar Nerve ....

Sub.Trochlear Node...

Axilla ....

Oedema ....

Lower-Symmetry ....

Hygiene...

Infection ....

Nails...

Oedema ....

Varicose Veins ....

BACK: Hygiene...

Deformity ....

Pain...

Oedema ....

OBSTETRICAL EXAMINATION

BREAST: Development...

Consistency ....

Symmetry...

Veins...

Areola ....

Primary...

Secondary..........

Montgomery's Tuberculosis..........

Nipples condition..........

Colostrum..........

Lumps..........

Axillary Nodes..........

PERINEUM: Hygiene..........

Discharge..........

Bleeding..........

Pruritis..........

Infection..........

Oedema..........

Complaints if any..........

ABDOMEN

Measurements:

Fundal Height.......... cms

Abdominal Girth.......... cm

Gestational Age (by date)..........

Inspection:

Shape..........

Size..........

Hygiene..........

Scars..........

Veins..........

Fetal Movements..........

Linea Nigra..........

Striae..........

Palpation:

Fundal Palpation..........

Rt. Lateral..........

Lt. Lateral..........

Pelvic Palpation..........

Pawlick Grip..........

Ausculation:

FHS..........

Conclusion:

Lie..........

Attitude..........

Presentation..........

Position..........

Prest. Part: Eng/Not Engaged..........

INVESTIGATION

INVESTIGATION BIOCHEMICAL										BIOPHYSICAL						
S. No.	Date	Blood					Urine		Stool	USG						
		Hb	Blood Group	HIV	VDRL	Blood Sugar	R	C		NST	BPP	FL/CRL	Placenta	Gest.Wks	LIQ	Anamoly

Any Other: ....

Treatment: Drugs..........

Supportive: ....

DAILY OBSERVATION

Date	Temp	Pulse	Resp	BP	Weight	FSH	Urine output	Urine		Fundal HT	Abd. Girth	Kicks Count 4 hrly
								Albu	Sugar			

NURSING PROBLEM AND RELATED OBJECTIVE OF CARE

Actual Problem Nursing Problem..........

....

....

....

....

....

Potential Problem Nursing Problem..........

....

....

....

....

....

NURSING CARE PLAN

ASSESSMENT	NSG DIAGNOSIS	GOAL	PLANNING	IMPLEMENTATION

HEALTH EDUCATION

Date ....Topic..

Content

....

....

....

....

....

Teacher Signature...

ANTENATAL CARE STUDY

IDENTIFICATION DATA

Name of Mother..

Reg. No:..

Age: ....

Gravida: ....

Para:..

Diagnosis: ....

Date of Admission:..

Date of Discharge: ....

PAST MENSTRUAL HISTORY

LMP ....EDD ....Cycle..

HEALTH HISTORY

1. Past Obstetrical History..

   ....

   ....

2. Present Pregnancy History

   - I-trimester..

     ....

     ....

   - II-trimester..

     ....

     ....

- III-trimester...
....
....

3. Past Medical History...
....
....

4. Present Surgical History. ....
....
....

5. Past Surgical History. ....
....
....

6. Family History. ....
....
....

7. Personal History. ....
....
....

OBSTETRICAL HISTORY

S.No.	Year	Abortion	Prem	F.T.	Type of Labour and Mode of Delivery	Gender	Live or Still Birth	Remark

ANTENATAL ATTENDANCES

LMP............................ EDD..Gestation at 1st visit.................. wk

Date	Wt	BP	FHS	Weeks	Fundal Height	Presentation	Treatments and Remarks

GENERAL EXAMINATION

Poor/Fair/Good

Height: .... cms Weight:............................ Kgs

BP: mm Hg .... Temp: ....Pulse:..................... /Min Resp:......................../Min

Urine: Alb .... Sugar...

PHYSICAL EXAMINATION

HEAD: Hygiene..

Injury..

Surgery..

Infection ....

Any other ....

FACE: Expression..

Symmetry..

Chloasma ....

Scar..

EYES: Field of Vision..

Vision ....

Conjunctiva ....

Sclera. ....

Periorbital Oedema ....

Complaints if any ....

EARS: Hygiene..........

Hearing..........

Pain..........

Wax..........

Discharge..........

Surgery..........

Complaints if any..........

NOSE: Septal Deviation..........

Discharge..........

Bleeding..........

Polyp..........

Hygiene..........

Complaints if any..........

MOUTH: Lips: Colour.......... Texture..........

Stomatitis:..........

Hygiene:..........

Halitosis:..........

Tongue:..........

Teeth: Stain..........Symmetry..........Caries..........Extractions..........

Pain..........Fillings...........

GUMS: Colour..........

Bleeding..........

Gingivitis..........

Complaints if any..........

NECK: Hygiene..........

Nodes..........

Glands..........

Thyroid..........

Jugular Veins..........

Scar..........

Complaints if any..........

CHEST: Shape...

Scar. ....

LIMBS: Upper-Symmetry...

Tremors ....

Nails...

Hygiene...

Infection ....

Ulnar Nerve ....

Sub.Trochlear Node...

Axilla ....

Oedema ....

Lower-Symmetry ....

Hygiene...

Infection ....

Nails...

Oedema ....

Varicose Veins ....

BACK: Hygiene...

Deformity...

Pain...

Oedema ....

OBSTETRICAL EXAMINATION

BREAST: Development ....

Consistency ....

Symmetry...

Veins...

Areola ....

Primary...

Secondary ....

Montgomery's Tuberculosis ....

Nipples condition..........

Colostrum ....

Lumps..........

Axillary Nodes..........

PERINEUM: Hygiene..........

Discharge ....

Bleeding..........

Pruritis ....

Infection..........

Oedema ....

Complaints if any..........

ABDOMEN

Measurements:

Fundal Height.......... cms

Abdominal Girth.......... cm

Gestational Age (by date)..........

Inspection:

Shape..........

Size ....

Hygiene..........

Scars ....

Veins..........

Fetal Movements..........

Linea Nigra..........

Striae..........

Palpation:

Fundal Palpation..

Rt. Lateral..

Lt. Lateral..

Pelvic Palpation..

Pawlick Grip..

Ausculation:

FHS..

Conclusion:

Lie..

Attitude..

Presentation..

Position..

Prest. Part: Eng/Not Engaged..

INVESTIGATION

INVESTIGATION BIOCHEMICAL										BIOPHYSICAL							
S. No.	Date	Blood					Urine		Stool	USG							
		Hb	Blood Group	HIV	VDRL	Blood Sugar	R	C		NST	BPP	FL/CRL	Placenta	Gest.Wks	LIQ	Anamoly

Any Other: ....

Treatment: Drugs..

Supportive: ....

DAILY OBSERVATION

Date	Temp	Pulse	Resp	BP	Weight	FSH	Urine output	Urine		Fundal HT	Abd. Girth	Kicks Count 4 hrly
								Albu	Sugar			

NURSING PROBLEM AND RELATED OBJECTIVE OF CARE

Actual Problem Nursing Problem..

....

....

....

....

....

Potential Problem Nursing Problem...

....

....

....

....

....

NURSING CARE PLAN

ASSESSMENT	NSG DIAGNOSIS	GOAL	PLANNING	IMPLEMENTATION

HEALTH EDUCATION

Date ....Topic..

Content

....

....

....

....

....

Teacher Signature..

ANTENATAL CARE STUDY

IDENTIFICATION DATA

Name of Mother..

Reg. No:..

Age: ....

Gravida: ....

Para:..

Diagnosis: ....

Date of Admission:..

Date of Discharge: ....

PAST MENSTRUAL HISTORY

LMP ....EDD ....Cycle...

HEALTH HISTORY

1. Past Obstetrical History...

   ....

   ....

2. Present Pregnancy History

   - I-trimester ....

     ....

     ....

   - II-trimester...

     ....

     ....

- III-trimester..

....

....

3. Past Medical History..

....

....

4. Present Surgical History. ....

....

....

5. Past Surgical History. ....

....

....

6. Family History. ....

....

....

7. Personal History. ....

....

....

OBSTETRICAL HISTORY

S.No.	Year	Abortion	Prem	F.T.	Type of Labour and Mode of Delivery	Gender	Live or Still Birth	Remark

ANTENATAL ATTENDANCES

LMP.............................. EDD..Gestation at 1st visit................... wk

Date	Wt	BP	FHS	Weeks	Fundal Height	Presentation	Treatments and Remarks

GENERAL EXAMINATION

Poor/Fair/Good

Height: .... cms Weight:..........................Kgs

BP: mm Hg .... Temp: ....Pulse:..................... /Min Resp:......................./Min

Urine: Alb .... Sugar...

PHYSICAL EXAMINATION

HEAD: Hygiene...

Injury...

Surgery...

Infection ....

Any other ....

FACE: Expression...

Symmetry...

Chloasma ....

Scar...

EYES: Field of Vision...

Vision ....

Conjunctiva ....

Sclera. ....

Periorbital Oedema ....

Complaints if any ....

EARS: Hygiene..

Hearing..

Pain..

Wax..

Discharge..

Surgery..

Complaints if any..

NOSE: Septal Deviation..

Discharge..

Bleeding..

Polyp..

Hygiene..

Complaints if any..

MOUTH: Lips: Colour.................................... Texture....................................

Stomatitis:..

Hygiene:..

Halitosis:..

Tongue:..

Teeth: Stain..............................Symmetry.................. Caries..............................Extractions.....................

Pain ....Fillings. ....

GUMS: Colour..

Bleeding..

Gingivitis..

Complaints if any..

NECK: Hygiene..

Nodes..

Glands..

Thyroid..

Jugular Veins..

Scar..

Complaints if any..

CHEST: Shape...

Scar. ....

LIMBS: Upper-Symmetry...

Tremors...

Nails...

Hygiene...

Infection ....

Ulnar Nerve ....

Sub.Trochlear Node...

Axilla ....

Oedema...

Lower-Symmetry...

Hygiene...

Infection ....

Nails...

Oedema...

Varicose Veins...

BACK: Hygiene...

Deformity...

Pain...

Oedema...

OBSTETRICAL EXAMINATION

BREAST: Development...

Consistency ....

Symmetry...

Veins...

Areola ....

Primary...

Secondary ....

Montgomery's Tuberculosis ....

Nipples condition..

Colostrum ....

Lumps..

Axillary Nodes..

PERINEUM: Hygiene..

Discharge ....

Bleeding..

Pruritis ....

Infection..

Oedema ....

Complaints if any..

ABDOMEN

Measurements:

Fundal Height...cms

Abdominal Girth... cm

Gestational Age (by date)...

Inspection:

Shape..

Size ....

Hygiene..

Scars ....

Veins..

Fetal Movements..

Linea Nigra..

Striae ....

Palpation:

Fundal Palpation...

Rt. Lateral...

Lt. Lateral...

Pelvic Palpation...

Pawlick Grip...

Ausculation:

FHS...

Conclusion:

Lie...

Attitude...

Presentation...

Position...

Prest. Part: Eng/Not Engaged...

INVESTIGATION

INVESTIGATION BIOCHEMICAL										BIOPHYSICAL							
		Blood					Urine			USG							
S. No.	Date	Hb	Blood Group	HIV	VDRL	Blood Sugar	R	C	Stool	NST	BPP	FL/CRL	Placenta	Gest.Wks	LIQ	Anamoly	

Any Other: ....

Treatment: Drugs...

Supportive: ....

DAILY OBSERVATION

Date	Temp	Pulse	Resp	BP	Weight	FSH	Urine output	Urine		Fundal HT	Abd. Girth	Kicks Count 4 hrly
								Albu	Sugar			

NURSING PROBLEM AND RELATED OBJECTIVE OF CARE

Actual Problem Nursing Problem..

....

....

....

....

....

Potential Problem Nursing Problem..

....

....

....

....

....

NURSING CARE PLAN

ASSESSMENT	NSG DIAGNOSIS	GOAL	PLANNING	IMPLEMENTATION

HEALTH EDUCATION

Date ....Topic...

Content

....

....

....

....

....

Teacher Signature...

ANTENATAL CARE STUDY

IDENTIFICATION DATA

Name of Mother...

Reg. No:...

Age: ....

Gravida: ....

Para:...

Diagnosis: ....

Date of Admission:...

Date of Discharge: ....

PAST MENSTRUAL HISTORY

LMP ....EDD ....Cycle...

HEALTH HISTORY

1. Past Obstetrical History...

   ....

   ....

2. Present Pregnancy History

   - I-trimester ....

     ....

     ....

   - II-trimester...

     ....

     ....

- III-trimester...
    ....
    ....

3. Past Medical History...
    ....
    ....

4. Present Surgical History. ....
    ....
    ....

5. Past Surgical History...
    ....
    ....

6. Family History. ....
    ....
    ....

7. Personal History. ....
    ....
    ....

OBSTETRICAL HISTORY

S.No.	Year	Abortion	Prem	F.T.	Type of Labour and Mode of Delivery	Gender	Live or Still Birth	Remark

ANTENATAL ATTENDANCES

LMP............................. EDD..Gestation at 1st visit.................. wk

Date	Wt	BP	FHS	Weeks	Fundal Height	Presentation	Treatments and Remarks

GENERAL EXAMINATION

Poor/Fair/Good

Height: .... cms Weight:............................ Kgs

BP: mm Hg .... Temp: ....Pulse:..................... /Min Resp:......................./Min

Urine: Alb .... Sugar...

PHYSICAL EXAMINATION

HEAD: Hygiene...

Injury...

Surgery...

Infection ....

Any other ....

FACE: Expression...

Symmetry...

Chloasma ....

Scar...

EYES: Field of Vision...

Vision ....

Conjunctiva...

Sclera. ....

Periorbital Oedema ....

Complaints if any ....

EARS: Hygiene..

Hearing..

Pain..

Wax..

Discharge..

Surgery..

Complaints if any..

NOSE: Septal Deviation..

Discharge..

Bleeding..

Polyp..

Hygiene..

Complaints if any..

MOUTH: Lips: Colour.. Texture..

Stomatitis:..

Hygiene:..

Halitosis:..

Tongue:..

Teeth: Stain ....Symmetry........................ Caries..Extractions........................

Pain ....Fillings. ....

GUMS: Colour..

Bleeding..

Gingivitis..

Complaints if any..

NECK: Hygiene..

Nodes..

Glands..

Thyroid..

Jugular Veins..

Scar..

Complaints if any..

CHEST: Shape..

Scar. ....

LIMBS: Upper-Symmetry..

Tremors..

Nails..

Hygiene..

Infection ....

Ulnar Nerve ....

Sub.Trochlear Node..

Axilla ....

Oedema..

Lower-Symmetry..

Hygiene..

Infection ....

Nails..

Oedema..

Varicose Veins..

BACK: Hygiene..

Deformity..

Pain..

Oedema..

OBSTETRICAL EXAMINATION

BREAST: Development..

Consistency ....

Symmetry..

Veins..

Areola ....

Primary..

Secondary ....

Montgomery's Tuberculosis ....

Nipples condition..

Colostrum ....

Lumps..

Axillary Nodes...

PERINEUM: Hygiene...

Discharge ....

Bleeding...

Pruritis ....

Infection...

Oedema ....

Complaints if any..

ABDOMEN

Measurements:

Fundal Height... cms

Abdominal Girth.. cm

Gestational Age (by date)...

Inspection:

Shape...

Size ....

Hygiene...

Scars ....

Veins..

Fetal Movements...

Linea Nigra..

Striae ....

Palpation:

Fundal Palpation..........

Rt. Lateral..........

Lt. Lateral..........

Pelvic Palpation..........

Pawlick Grip..........

Ausculation:

FHS..........

Conclusion:

Lie..........

Attitude..........

Presentation..........

Position..........

Prest. Part: Eng/Not Engaged..........

INVESTIGATION

INVESTIGATION BIOCHEMICAL											BIOPHYSICAL						
		Blood					Urine			USG							
S. No.	Date	Hb	Blood Group	HIV	VDRL	Blood Sugar	R	C	Stool	NST	BPP	FL/CRL	Placenta	Gest.Wks	LIQ	Anamoly

Any Other: ....

Treatment: Drugs..........

Supportive: ....

DAILY OBSERVATION

Date	Temp	Pulse	Resp	BP	Weight	FSH	Urine output	Urine		Fundal HT	Abd. Girth	Kicks Count 4 hrly
								Albu	Sugar			

NURSING PROBLEM AND RELATED OBJECTIVE OF CARE

Actual Problem Nursing Problem..

....

....

....

....

....

Potential Problem Nursing Problem..

....

....

....

....

....

NURSING CARE PLAN

ASSESSMENT	NSG DIAGNOSIS	GOAL	PLANNING	IMPLEMENTATION

HEALTH EDUCATION

Date ....Topic..

Content

....

....

....

....

....

Teacher Signature..

ANTENATAL CARE STUDY

IDENTIFICATION DATA

Name of Mother..

Reg. No:..

Age: ....

Gravida: ....

Para:..

Diagnosis: ....

Date of Admission:..

Date of Discharge: ....

PAST MENSTRUAL HISTORY

LMP ....EDD ....Cycle..

HEALTH HISTORY

1. Past Obstetrical History..

   ....

   ....

2. Present Pregnancy History

   - I-trimester ....

     ....

     ....

   - II-trimester..

     ....

     ....

- III-trimester..

   ....

   ....

3. Past Medical History ....

   ....

   ....

4. Present Surgical History. ....

   ....

   ....

5. Past Surgical History. ....

   ....

   ....

6. Family History. ....

   ....

   ....

7. Personal History. ....

   ....

   ....

OBSTETRICAL HISTORY

S.No.	Year	Abortion	Prem	F.T.	Type of Labour and Mode of Delivery	Gender	Live or Still Birth	Remark

ANTENATAL ATTENDANCES

LMP............................ EDD...Gestation at 1st visit.................. wk

Date	Wt	BP	FHS	Weeks	Fundal Height	Presentation	Treatments and Remarks

GENERAL EXAMINATION

Poor/Fair/Good

Height: .... cms Weight:............................Kgs

BP: mm Hg .... Temp: ....Pulse:..................... /Min Resp:......................./Min

Urine: Alb .... Sugar...

PHYSICAL EXAMINATION

HEAD: Hygiene...

Injury...

Surgery...

Infection ....

Any other ....

FACE: Expression...

Symmetry...

Chloasma ....

Scar...

EYES: Field of Vision...

Vision ....

Conjunctiva ....

Sclera. ....

Periorbital Oedema ....

Complaints if any ....

EARS: Hygiene...

Hearing...

Pain...

Wax...

Discharge...

Surgery...

Complaints if any...

NOSE: Septal Deviation...

Discharge...

Bleeding...

Polyp...

Hygiene...

Complaints if any...

MOUTH: Lips: Colour.................................... Texture....................................

Stomatitis:...

Hygiene:...

Halitosis:...

Tongue:...

Teeth: Stain................................Symmetry..................Caries..............................Extractions.......................

Pain ....Fillings. ....

GUMS: Colour...

Bleeding...

Gingivitis...

Complaints if any...

NECK: Hygiene...

Nodes...

Glands...

Thyroid...

Jugular Veins...

Scar...

Complaints if any...

CHEST: Shape...

Scar. ....

LIMBS: Upper-Symmetry...

Tremors...

Nails...

Hygiene...

Infection ....

Ulnar Nerve ....

Sub.Trochlear Node...

Axilla ....

Oedema...

Lower-Symmetry...

Hygiene...

Infection ....

Nails...

Oedema...

Varicose Veins...

BACK: Hygiene...

Deformity...

Pain...

Oedema...

OBSTETRICAL EXAMINATION

BREAST: Development...

Consistency ....

Symmetry...

Veins...

Areola ....

Primary...

Secondary ....

Montgomery's Tuberculosis ....

Nipples condition ....

Colostrum ....

Lumps ....

Axillary Nodes ....

PERINEUM: Hygiene ....

Discharge ....

Bleeding ....

Pruritis ....

Infection ....

Oedema ....

Complaints if any ....

ABDOMEN

Measurements:

Fundal Height .... cms

Abdominal Girth .... cm

Gestational Age (by date) ....

Inspection:

Shape ....

Size ....

Hygiene ....

Scars ....

Veins ....

Fetal Movements ....

Linea Nigra ....

Striae ....

Palpation:

Fundal Palpation..

Rt. Lateral..

Lt. Lateral..

Pelvic Palpation..

Pawlick Grip..

Ausculation:

FHS..

Conclusion:

Lie..

Attitude..

Presentation..

Position..

Prest. Part: Eng/Not Engaged..

INVESTIGATION

INVESTIGATION BIOCHEMICAL										BIOPHYSICAL						
S. No.	Date	Blood					Urine		Stool	USG						
		Hb	Blood Group	HIV	VDRL	Blood Sugar	R	C		NST	BPP	FL/CRL	Placenta	Gest.Wks	LIQ	Anamoly

Any Other: ....

Treatment: Drugs..

Supportive: ....

DAILY OBSERVATION

Date	Temp	Pulse	Resp	BP	Weight	FSH	Urine output	Urine		Fundal HT	Abd. Girth	Kicks Count 4 hrly
								Albu	Sugar			

NURSING PROBLEM AND RELATED OBJECTIVE OF CARE

Actual Problem Nursing Problem...

....

....

....

....

....

Potential Problem Nursing Problem...

....

....

....

....

....

NURSING CARE PLAN

ASSESSMENT	NSG DIAGNOSIS	GOAL	PLANNING	IMPLEMENTATION

HEALTH EDUCATION

Date ....Topic...

Content

....

....

....

....

....

Teacher Signature..

ANTENATAL CARE STUDY

IDENTIFICATION DATA

Name of Mother..

Reg. No:...

Age: ....

Gravida: ....

Para:...

Diagnosis: ....

Date of Admission:...

Date of Discharge: ....

PAST MENSTRUAL HISTORY

LMP .... EDD .... Cycle...

HEALTH HISTORY

1. Past Obstetrical History...

   ....

   ....

2. Present Pregnancy History

   - I-trimester ....

     ....

     ....

   - II-trimester ....

     ....

     ....

- III-trimester..
....
....

3. Past Medical History..
....
....

4. Present Surgical History...
....
....

5. Past Surgical History...
....
....

6. Family History...
....
....

7. Personal History...
....
....

OBSTETRICAL HISTORY

S.No.	Year	Abortion	Prem	F.T.	Type of Labour and Mode of Delivery	Gender	Live or Still Birth	Remark

ANTENATAL ATTENDANCES

LMP............................ EDD..Gestation at 1st visit.................. wk

Date	Wt	BP	FHS	Weeks	Fundal Height	Presentation	Treatments and Remarks

GENERAL EXAMINATION

Poor/Fair/Good

Height: .... cms Weight:............................Kgs

BP: mm Hg .... Temp: ....Pulse:..................... /Min Resp:......................./Min

Urine: Alb .... Sugar...

PHYSICAL EXAMINATION

HEAD: Hygiene...

Injury...

Surgery...

Infection ....

Any other ....

FACE: Expression...

Symmetry...

Chloasma ....

Scar...

EYES: Field of Vision...

Vision ....

Conjunctiva ....

Sclera. ....

Periorbital Oedema ....

Complaints if any ....

EARS: Hygiene..........

Hearing..........

Pain..........

Wax..........

Discharge..........

Surgery..........

Complaints if any..........

NOSE: Septal Deviation..........

Discharge..........

Bleeding..........

Polyp..........

Hygiene..........

Complaints if any..........

MOUTH: Lips: Colour.......... Texture..........

Stomatitis:..........

Hygiene:..........

Halitosis:..........

Tongue:..........

Teeth: Stain..........Symmetry..........Caries..........Extractions..........

Pain..........Fillings...........

GUMS: Colour..........

Bleeding..........

Gingivitis..........

Complaints if any..........

NECK: Hygiene..........

Nodes..........

Glands..........

Thyroid..........

Jugular Veins..........

Scar..........

Complaints if any..........

CHEST: Shape..

Scar. ....

LIMBS: Upper-Symmetry..

Tremors..

Nails..

Hygiene..

Infection ....

Ulnar Nerve ....

Sub.Trochlear Node..

Axilla ....

Oedema..

Lower-Symmetry..

Hygiene..

Infection ....

Nails..

Oedema..

Varicose Veins..

BACK: Hygiene..

Deformity..

Pain..

Oedema..

OBSTETRICAL EXAMINATION

BREAST: Development..

Consistency ....

Symmetry..

Veins..

Areola ....

Primary..

Secondary ....

Montgomery's Tuberculosis ....

Nipples condition...

Colostrum ....

Lumps..

Axillary Nodes...

PERINEUM: Hygiene...

Discharge ....

Bleeding...

Pruritis ....

Infection...

Oedema ....

Complaints if any...

ABDOMEN

Measurements:

Fundal Height.. cms

Abdominal Girth... cm

Gestational Age (by date)..

Inspection:

Shape...

Size ....

Hygiene..

Scars ....

Veins..

Fetal Movements...

Linea Nigra...

Striae ....

Palpation:

Fundal Palpation..........

Rt. Lateral..........

Lt. Lateral..........

Pelvic Palpation..........

Pawlick Grip..........

Ausculation:

FHS..........

Conclusion:

Lie..........

Attitude..........

Presentation..........

Position..........

Prest. Part: Eng/Not Engaged..........

INVESTIGATION

INVESTIGATION BIOCHEMICAL										BIOPHYSICAL						
S. No.	Date	Blood					Urine		Stool	USG						
		Hb	Blood Group	HIV	VDRL	Blood Sugar	R	C		NST	BPP	FL/CRL	Placenta	Gest.Wks	LIQ	Anamoly

Any Other: ....

Treatment: Drugs..........

Supportive: ....

DAILY OBSERVATION

Date	Temp	Pulse	Resp	BP	Weight	FSH	Urine output	Urine		Fundal HT	Abd. Girth	Kicks Count 4 hrly
								Albu	Sugar			

NURSING PROBLEM AND RELATED OBJECTIVE OF CARE

Actual Problem Nursing Problem..

....

....

....

....

....

Potential Problem Nursing Problem..

....

....

....

....

....

NURSING CARE PLAN

ASSESSMENT	NSG DIAGNOSIS	GOAL	PLANNING	IMPLEMENTATION

HEALTH EDUCATION

Date ....Topic..

Content

....

....

....

....

....

Teacher Signature..

ANTENATAL CARE STUDY

IDENTIFICATION DATA

Name of Mother..

Reg. No:..

Age: ....

Gravida: ....

Para:..

Diagnosis: ....

Date of Admission:..

Date of Discharge: ....

PAST MENSTRUAL HISTORY

LMP ....EDD ....Cycle..

HEALTH HISTORY

1. Past Obstetrical History..

   ....

   ....

2. Present Pregnancy History

   - I-trimester ....

     ....

     ....

   - II-trimester..

     ....

     ....

- III-trimester...
....
....

3. Past Medical History...
....
....

4. Present Surgical History. ....
....
....

5. Past Surgical History. ....
....
....

6. Family History. ....
....
....

7. Personal History. ....
....
....

OBSTETRICAL HISTORY

S.No.	Year	Abortion	Prem	F.T.	Type of Labour and Mode of Delivery	Gender	Live or Still Birth	Remark

ANTENATAL ATTENDANCES

LMP............................ EDD..Gestation at 1st visit.................. wk

Date	Wt	BP	FHS	Weeks	Fundal Height	Presentation	Treatments and Remarks

GENERAL EXAMINATION

Poor/Fair/Good

Height: .... cms Weight:........................... Kgs

BP: mm Hg .... Temp: ....Pulse:..................... /Min Resp:......................./Min

Urine: Alb .... Sugar..

PHYSICAL EXAMINATION

HEAD: Hygiene...

Injury...

Surgery...

Infection ....

Any other ....

FACE: Expression...

Symmetry...

Chloasma ....

Scar...

EYES: Field of Vision...

Vision ....

Conjunctiva ....

Sclera. ....

Periorbital Oedema ....

Complaints if any ....

EARS: Hygiene..

Hearing ....

Pain..

Wax..

Discharge ....

Surgery..

Complaints if any ....

NOSE: Septal Deviation ....

Discharge ....

Bleeding ....

Polyp ....

Hygiene..

Complaints if any ....

MOUTH: Lips: Colour....................................... Texture ....

Stomatitis: ....

Hygiene: ....

Halitosis: ....

Tongue: ....

Teeth: Stain.................................Symmetry.................... Caries................................Extractions ....

Pain ....Fillings. ....

GUMS: Colour..

Bleeding ....

Gingivitis ....

Complaints if any ....

NECK: Hygiene..

Nodes ....

Glands ....

Thyroid ....

Jugular Veins ....

Scar..

Complaints if any ....

CHEST: Shape............

Scar. ....

LIMBS: Upper-Symmetry............

Tremors............

Nails............

Hygiene............

Infection ....

Ulnar Nerve ....

Sub.Trochlear Node............

Axilla ....

Oedema............

Lower-Symmetry............

Hygiene............

Infection ....

Nails............

Oedema............

Varicose Veins............

BACK: Hygiene............

Deformity............

Pain............

Oedema............

OBSTETRICAL EXAMINATION

BREAST: Development............

Consistency ....

Symmetry............

Veins............

Areola ....

Primary............

Secondary ....

Montgomery's Tuberculosis ....

Nipples condition ....

Colostrum ....

Lumps ....

Axillary Nodes ....

PERINEUM: Hygiene ....

Discharge ....

Bleeding ....

Pruritis ....

Infection ....

Oedema ....

Complaints if any ....

ABDOMEN

Measurements:

Fundal Height .... cms

Abdominal Girth .... cm

Gestational Age (by date) ....

Inspection:

Shape ....

Size ....

Hygiene ....

Scars ....

Veins ....

Fetal Movements ....

Linea Nigra ....

Striae ....

Palpation:

Fundal Palpation..........

Rt. Lateral..........

Lt. Lateral..........

Pelvic Palpation..........

Pawlick Grip..........

Ausculation:

FHS..........

Conclusion:

Lie..........

Attitude..........

Presentation..........

Position..........

Prest. Part: Eng/Not Engaged..........

INVESTIGATION

INVESTIGATION BIOCHEMICAL											BIOPHYSICAL						
		Blood					Urine			USG							
S. No.	Date	Hb	Blood Group	HIV	VDRL	Blood Sugar	R	C	Stool	NST	BPP	FL/CRL	Placenta	Gest.Wks	LIQ	Anamoly

Any Other: ....

Treatment: Drugs..........

Supportive: ....

DAILY OBSERVATION

Date	Temp	Pulse	Resp	BP	Weight	FSH	Urine output	Urine		Fundal HT	Abd. Girth	Kicks Count 4 hrly
								Albu	Sugar			

NURSING PROBLEM AND RELATED OBJECTIVE OF CARE

Actual Problem Nursing Problem..........

Potential Problem Nursing Problem..........

NURSING CARE PLAN

ASSESSMENT	NSG DIAGNOSIS	GOAL	PLANNING	IMPLEMENTATION

HEALTH EDUCATION

Date ....Topic...

Content

....

....

....

....

....

Teacher Signature...

ANTENATAL CARE STUDY

IDENTIFICATION DATA

Name of Mother...

Reg. No:..

Age: ....

Gravida: ....

Para:..

Diagnosis: ....

Date of Admission:..

Date of Discharge: ....

PAST MENSTRUAL HISTORY

LMP ....EDD ....Cycle...

HEALTH HISTORY

1. Past Obstetrical History...

   ....

   ....

2. Present Pregnancy History

   - I-trimester ....

     ....

     ....

   - II-trimester...

     ....

     ....

- III-trimester..

....

....

3. Past Medical History..

....

....

4. Present Surgical History. ....

....

....

5. Past Surgical History. ....

....

....

6. Family History. ....

....

....

7. Personal History. ....

....

....

OBSTETRICAL HISTORY

S.No.	Year	Abortion	Prem	F.T.	Type of Labour and Mode of Delivery	Gender	Live or Still Birth	Remark

ANTENATAL ATTENDANCES

LMP............................ EDD.......................................Gestation at 1st visit.................. wk

Date	Wt	BP	FHS	Weeks	Fundal Height	Presentation	Treatments and Remarks

GENERAL EXAMINATION

Poor/Fair/Good

Height: .... cms Weight:............................Kgs

BP: mm Hg .... Temp: ....Pulse:...................... /Min Resp:......................../Min

Urine: Alb .... Sugar ....

PHYSICAL EXAMINATION

HEAD: Hygiene..

Injury..

Surgery..

Infection ....

Any other ....

FACE: Expression..

Symmetry..

Chloasma ....

Scar..

EYES: Field of Vision..

Vision ....

Conjunctiva ....

Sclera. ....

Periorbital Oedema ....

Complaints if any ....

EARS: Hygiene..........

Hearing..........

Pain..........

Wax..........

Discharge..........

Surgery..........

Complaints if any..........

NOSE: Septal Deviation..........

Discharge..........

Bleeding..........

Polyp..........

Hygiene..........

Complaints if any..........

MOUTH: Lips: Colour.......... Texture..........

Stomatitis:..........

Hygiene:..........

Halitosis:..........

Tongue:..........

Teeth: Stain..........Symmetry.......... Caries..........Extractions..........

Pain ....Fillings. ....

GUMS: Colour..........

Bleeding..........

Gingivitis..........

Complaints if any..........

NECK: Hygiene..........

Nodes..........

Glands..........

Thyroid..........

Jugular Veins..........

Scar..........

Complaints if any..........

CHEST: Shape..

Scar. ....

LIMBS: Upper-Symmetry..

Tremors..

Nails..

Hygiene..

Infection ....

Ulnar Nerve ....

Sub.Trochlear Node..

Axilla ....

Oedema..

Lower-Symmetry..

Hygiene..

Infection ....

Nails..

Oedema..

Varicose Veins..

BACK: Hygiene..

Deformity..

Pain..

Oedema..

OBSTETRICAL EXAMINATION

BREAST: Development..

Consistency ....

Symmetry..

Veins..

Areola ....

Primary..

Secondary ....

Montgomery's Tuberculosis ....

Nipples condition...

Colostrum ....

Lumps...

Axillary Nodes...

PERINEUM: Hygiene...

Discharge ....

Bleeding..

Pruritis ....

Infection..

Oedema ....

Complaints if any..

ABDOMEN

Measurements:

Fundal Height..cms

Abdominal Girth.. cm

Gestational Age (by date)...

Inspection:

Shape ....

Size ....

Hygiene...

Scars ....

Veins...

Fetal Movements..

Linea Nigra...

Striae ....

Palpation:

Fundal Palpation...

Rt. Lateral...

Lt. Lateral...

Pelvic Palpation...

Pawlick Grip...

Ausculation:

FHS...

Conclusion:

Lie...

Attitude...

Presentation...

Position...

Prest. Part: Eng/Not Engaged...

INVESTIGATION

INVESTIGATION BIOCHEMICAL										BIOPHYSICAL							
		Blood					Urine			USG							
S. No.	Date	Hb	Blood Group	HIV	VDRL	Blood Sugar	R	C	Stool	NST	BPP	FL/CRL	Placenta	Gest.Wks	LIQ	Anamoly

Any Other: ....

Treatment: Drugs...

Supportive: ....

DAILY OBSERVATION

Date	Temp	Pulse	Resp	BP	Weight	FSH	Urine output	Urine		Fundal HT	Abd. Girth	Kicks Count 4 hrly
								Albu	Sugar			

NURSING PROBLEM AND RELATED OBJECTIVE OF CARE

Actual Problem Nursing Problem..

....

....

....

....

....

Potential Problem Nursing Problem..

....

....

....

....

....

NURSING CARE PLAN

ASSESSMENT	NSG DIAGNOSIS	GOAL	PLANNING	IMPLEMENTATION

HEALTH EDUCATION

Date ....Topic..

Content

....

....

....

....

....

Teacher Signature...

ANTENATAL CARE STUDY

IDENTIFICATION DATA

Name of Mother...

Reg. No:...

Age: ....

Gravida: ....

Para:...

Diagnosis: ....

Date of Admission:..

Date of Discharge: ....

PAST MENSTRUAL HISTORY

LMP ....EDD ....Cycle...

HEALTH HISTORY

1. Past Obstetrical History..

   ....

   ....

2. Present Pregnancy History

   - I-trimester ....

     ....

     ....

   - II-trimester ....

     ....

     ....

- III-trimester..

  ....

  ....

3. Past Medical History..

   ....

   ....

4. Present Surgical History. ....

   ....

   ....

5. Past Surgical History. ....

   ....

   ....

6. Family History. ....

   ....

   ....

7. Personal History. ....

   ....

   ....

OBSTETRICAL HISTORY

S.No.	Year	Abortion	Prem	F.T.	Type of Labour and Mode of Delivery	Gender	Live or Still Birth	Remark

ANTENATAL ATTENDANCES

LMP............................ EDD...Gestation at 1st visit.................. wk

Date	Wt	BP	FHS	Weeks	Fundal Height	Presentation	Treatments and Remarks

GENERAL EXAMINATION

Poor/Fair/Good

Height: .... cms Weight:........................... Kgs

BP: mm Hg .... Temp: ....Pulse:..................... /Min Resp:......................./Min

Urine: Alb .... Sugar..

PHYSICAL EXAMINATION

HEAD: Hygiene...

Injury...

Surgery...

Infection ....

Any other ....

FACE: Expression...

Symmetry...

Chloasma ....

Scar...

EYES: Field of Vision...

Vision ....

Conjunctiva ....

Sclera. ....

Periorbital Oedema ....

Complaints if any ....

EARS: Hygiene..

Hearing ....

Pain..

Wax..

Discharge ....

Surgery..

Complaints if any ....

NOSE: Septal Deviation ....

Discharge ....

Bleeding ....

Polyp ....

Hygiene..

Complaints if any ....

MOUTH: Lips: Colour...................................... Texture ....

Stomatitis:..

Hygiene:..

Halitosis: ....

Tongue: ....

Teeth: Stain..................................Symmetry.................... Caries................................Extractions ....

Pain ....Fillings. ....

GUMS: Colour..

Bleeding ....

Gingivitis ....

Complaints if any ....

NECK: Hygiene..

Nodes ....

Glands ....

Thyroid..

Jugular Veins..

Scar..

Complaints if any ....

CHEST: Shape............

Scar. ....

LIMBS: Upper-Symmetry............

Tremors............

Nails............

Hygiene............

Infection ....

Ulnar Nerve ....

Sub.Trochlear Node............

Axilla ....

Oedema............

Lower-Symmetry............

Hygiene............

Infection ....

Nails............

Oedema............

Varicose Veins............

BACK: Hygiene............

Deformity............

Pain............

Oedema............

OBSTETRICAL EXAMINATION

BREAST: Development............

Consistency ....

Symmetry............

Veins............

Areola ....

Primary............

Secondary ....

Montgomery's Tuberculosis ....

Nipples condition ....

Colostrum ....

Lumps ....

Axillary Nodes ....

PERINEUM: Hygiene ....

Discharge ....

Bleeding ....

Pruritis ....

Infection ....

Oedema ....

Complaints if any ....

ABDOMEN

Measurements:

Fundal Height .... cms

Abdominal Girth .... cm

Gestational Age (by date) ....

Inspection:

Shape ....

Size ....

Hygiene ....

Scars ....

Veins ....

Fetal Movements ....

Linea Nigra ....

Striae ....

Palpation:

Fundal Palpation..........

Rt. Lateral..........

Lt. Lateral..........

Pelvic Palpation..........

Pawlick Grip..........

Ausculation:

FHS..........

Conclusion:

Lie..........

Attitude..........

Presentation..........

Position..........

Prest. Part: Eng/Not Engaged..........

INVESTIGATION

INVESTIGATION BIOCHEMICAL										BIOPHYSICAL							
S. No.	Date	Blood					Urine		Stool	USG							
		Hb	Blood Group	HIV	VDRL	Blood Sugar	R	C		NST	BPP	FL/CRL	Placenta	Gest.Wks	LIQ	Anamoly

Any Other: ....

Treatment: Drugs..........

Supportive: ....

DAILY OBSERVATION

Date	Temp	Pulse	Resp	BP	Weight	FSH	Urine output	Urine		Fundal HT	Abd. Girth	Kicks Count 4 hrly
								Albu	Sugar			

NURSING PROBLEM AND RELATED OBJECTIVE OF CARE

Actual Problem Nursing Problem..

....

....

....

....

....

Potential Problem Nursing Problem..

....

....

....

....

....

NURSING CARE PLAN

ASSESSMENT	NSG DIAGNOSIS	GOAL	PLANNING	IMPLEMENTATION

HEALTH EDUCATION

Date ....Topic..

Content

....

....

....

....

....

Teacher Signature..

ANTENATAL CARE STUDY

IDENTIFICATION DATA

Name of Mother..

Reg. No:...

Age: ....

Gravida: ....

Para:...

Diagnosis: ....

Date of Admission:...

Date of Discharge: ....

PAST MENSTRUAL HISTORY

LMP ....EDD ....Cycle.......................................

HEALTH HISTORY

1. Past Obstetrical History...

 ....

 ....

2. Present Pregnancy History
   - I-trimester ....

     ....

     ....

   - II-trimester...

     ....

     ....

- III-trimester...

....

....

3. Past Medical History ....

....

....

4. Present Surgical History. ....

....

....

5. Past Surgical History. ....

....

....

6. Family History. ....

....

....

7. Personal History. ....

....

....

OBSTETRICAL HISTORY

S.No.	Year	Abortion	Prem	F.T.	Type of Labour and Mode of Delivery	Gender	Live or Still Birth	Remark

ANTENATAL ATTENDANCES

LMP............................. EDD...Gestation at 1st visit................... wk

Date	Wt	BP	FHS	Weeks	Fundal Height	Presentation	Treatments and Remarks

GENERAL EXAMINATION

Poor/Fair/Good

Height: .... cms Weight:............................Kgs

BP: mm Hg .... Temp: ....Pulse:..................... /Min Resp:........................./Min

Urine: Alb .... Sugar...

PHYSICAL EXAMINATION

HEAD: Hygiene...

Injury...

Surgery...

Infection ....

Any other ....

FACE: Expression...

Symmetry...

Chloasma ....

Scar...

EYES: Field of Vision...

Vision ....

Conjunctiva ....

Sclera. ....

Periorbital Oedema ....

Complaints if any ....

EARS: Hygiene..

Hearing..

Pain..

Wax..

Discharge..

Surgery..

Complaints if any..

NOSE: Septal Deviation..

Discharge..

Bleeding..

Polyp..

Hygiene..

Complaints if any..

MOUTH: Lips: Colour.................................... Texture....................................

Stomatitis:..

Hygiene:..

Halitosis:..

Tongue:..

Teeth: Stain.............................Symmetry...................Caries.............................Extractions......................

Pain ....Fillings. ....

GUMS: Colour..

Bleeding..

Gingivitis..

Complaints if any..

NECK: Hygiene..

Nodes..

Glands..

Thyroid..

Jugular Veins..

Scar..

Complaints if any..

CHEST: Shape..

Scar..

LIMBS: Upper-Symmetry..

Tremors..

Nails..

Hygiene..

Infection..

Ulnar Nerve..

Sub.Trochlear Node..

Axilla..

Oedema..

Lower-Symmetry..

Hygiene..

Infection..

Nails..

Oedema..

Varicose Veins..

BACK: Hygiene..

Deformity..

Pain..

Oedema..

OBSTETRICAL EXAMINATION

BREAST: Development..

Consistency..

Symmetry..

Veins..

Areola..

Primary..

Secondary ....

Montgomery's Tuberculosis ....

Nipples condition..

Colostrum ....

Lumps...

Axillary Nodes..

PERINEUM: Hygiene..

Discharge ....

Bleeding...

Pruritis ....

Infection...

Oedema ....

Complaints if any...

ABDOMEN

Measurements:

Fundal Height.. cms

Abdominal Girth.. cm

Gestational Age (by date)..

Inspection:

Shape...

Size ....

Hygiene...

Scars ....

Veins..

Fetal Movements..

Linea Nigra...

Striae..

Palpation:

Fundal Palpation..

Rt. Lateral..

Lt. Lateral..

Pelvic Palpation..

Pawlick Grip..

Ausculation:

FHS..

Conclusion:

Lie..

Attitude..

Presentation..

Position..

Prest. Part: Eng/Not Engaged..

INVESTIGATION

INVESTIGATION BIOCHEMICAL											BIOPHYSICAL					
		Blood					Urine			USG						
S. No.	Date	Hb	Blood Group	HIV	VDRL	Blood Sugar	R	C	Stool	NST	BPP	FL/CRL	Placenta	Gest.Wks	LIQ	Anamoly

Any Other: ....

Treatment: Drugs..

Supportive: ....

DAILY OBSERVATION

Date	Temp	Pulse	Resp	BP	Weight	FSH	Urine output	Urine		Fundal HT	Abd. Girth	Kicks Count 4 hrly
								Albu	Sugar			

NURSING PROBLEM AND RELATED OBJECTIVE OF CARE

Actual Problem Nursing Problem..

....

....

....

....

....

Potential Problem Nursing Problem..

....

....

....

....

....

NURSING CARE PLAN

ASSESSMENT	NSG DIAGNOSIS	GOAL	PLANNING	IMPLEMENTATION

HEALTH EDUCATION

Date ....Topic...

Content

....

....

....

....

....

Teacher Signature..

ANTENATAL CARE STUDY

IDENTIFICATION DATA

Name of Mother..

Reg. No:..

Age: ....

Gravida: ....

Para:..

Diagnosis: ....

Date of Admission:..

Date of Discharge: ....

PAST MENSTRUAL HISTORY

LMP ....EDD ....Cycle..

HEALTH HISTORY

1. Past Obstetrical History..

   ....

   ....

2. Present Pregnancy History
   - I-trimester..

     ....

     ....

   - II-trimester..

     ....

     ....

- III-trimester...

  ....

  ....

3. Past Medical History...

   ....

   ....

4. Present Surgical History. ....

   ....

   ....

5. Past Surgical History. ....

   ....

   ....

6. Family History. ....

   ....

   ....

7. Personal History. ....

   ....

   ....

OBSTETRICAL HISTORY

S.No.	Year	Abortion	Prem	F.T.	Type of Labour and Mode of Delivery	Gender	Live or Still Birth	Remark

ANTENATAL ATTENDANCES

LMP............................ EDD..Gestation at 1st visit.................. wk

Date	Wt	BP	FHS	Weeks	Fundal Height	Presentation	Treatments and Remarks

GENERAL EXAMINATION

Poor/Fair/Good

Height: .... cms Weight:............................ Kgs

BP: mm Hg .... Temp: ....Pulse:..................... /Min Resp:......................./Min

Urine: Alb .... Sugar...

PHYSICAL EXAMINATION

HEAD: Hygiene..

Injury..

Surgery..

Infection ....

Any other ....

FACE: Expression..

Symmetry..

Chloasma ....

Scar..

EYES: Field of Vision..

Vision ....

Conjunctiva ....

Sclera. ....

Periorbital Oedema ....

Complaints if any ....

EARS: Hygiene..

Hearing..

Pain..

Wax..

Discharge..

Surgery..

Complaints if any..

NOSE: Septal Deviation..

Discharge..

Bleeding..

Polyp..

Hygiene..

Complaints if any..

MOUTH: Lips: Colour.. Texture..

Stomatitis:..

Hygiene:..

Halitosis:..

Tongue:..

Teeth: Stain..................................Symmetry.................... Caries..................................Extractions.......................

Pain ....Fillings. ....

GUMS: Colour..

Bleeding..

Gingivitis..

Complaints if any..

NECK: Hygiene..

Nodes..

Glands..

Thyroid..

Jugular Veins..

Scar..

Complaints if any..

CHEST: Shape...

Scar. ....

LIMBS: Upper-Symmetry...

Tremors...

Nails...

Hygiene...

Infection ....

Ulnar Nerve ....

Sub.Trochlear Node...

Axilla ....

Oedema...

Lower-Symmetry...

Hygiene...

Infection ....

Nails...

Oedema...

Varicose Veins...

BACK: Hygiene...

Deformity...

Pain...

Oedema...

OBSTETRICAL EXAMINATION

BREAST: Development...

Consistency ....

Symmetry...

Veins...

Areola ....

Primary...

Secondary ....

Montgomery's Tuberculosis ....

Nipples condition ....

Colostrum ....

Lumps ....

Axillary Nodes ....

PERINEUM: Hygiene ....

Discharge ....

Bleeding ....

Pruritis ....

Infection ....

Oedema ....

Complaints if any ....

ABDOMEN

Measurements:

Fundal Height .... cms

Abdominal Girth .... cm

Gestational Age (by date) ....

Inspection:

Shape ....

Size ....

Hygiene ....

Scars ....

Veins ....

Fetal Movements ....

Linea Nigra ....

Striae ....

Palpation:

Fundal Palpation..

Rt. Lateral..

Lt. Lateral..

Pelvic Palpation..

Pawlick Grip..

Ausculation:

FHS..

Conclusion:

Lie..

Attitude..

Presentation..

Position ....

Prest. Part: Eng/Not Engaged..

INVESTIGATION

INVESTIGATION BIOCHEMICAL										BIOPHYSICAL							
		Blood					Urine			USG							
S. No.	Date	Hb	Blood Group	HIV	VDRL	Blood Sugar	R	C	Stool	NST	BPP	FL/CRL	Placenta	Gest.Wks	LIQ	Anamoly

Any Other: ....

Treatment: Drugs..

Supportive: ....

DAILY OBSERVATION

Date	Temp	Pulse	Resp	BP	Weight	FSH	Urine output	Urine		Fundal HT	Abd. Girth	Kicks Count 4 hrly
								Albu	Sugar			

NURSING PROBLEM AND RELATED OBJECTIVE OF CARE

Actual Problem Nursing Problem..

....

....

....

....

....

Potential Problem Nursing Problem..

....

....

....

....

....

NURSING CARE PLAN

ASSESSMENT	NSG DIAGNOSIS	GOAL	PLANNING	IMPLEMENTATION

HEALTH EDUCATION

Date ....Topic..

Content

....

....

....

....

....

Teacher Signature...

ANTENATAL CARE STUDY

IDENTIFICATION DATA

Name of Mother..

Reg. No:..

Age: ....

Gravida: ....

Para:..

Diagnosis: ....

Date of Admission:..

Date of Discharge: ....

PAST MENSTRUAL HISTORY

LMP .... EDD .... Cycle..

HEALTH HISTORY

1. Past Obstetrical History..

   ....

   ....

2. Present Pregnancy History

   - I-trimester..

     ....

     ....

   - II-trimester..

     ....

     ....

- III-trimester..

....

....

3. Past Medical History..

....

....

4. Present Surgical History...

....

....

5. Past Surgical History...

....

....

6. Family History...

....

....

7. Personal History...

....

....

OBSTETRICAL HISTORY

S.No.	Year	Abortion	Prem	F.T.	Type of Labour and Mode of Delivery	Gender	Live or Still Birth	Remark

ANTENATAL ATTENDANCES

LMP.............................. EDD...Gestation at 1st visit.................. wk

Date	Wt	BP	FHS	Weeks	Fundal Height	Presentation	Treatments and Remarks

GENERAL EXAMINATION

Poor/Fair/Good

Height: .... cms Weight:............................. Kgs

BP: mm Hg .... Temp: ....Pulse:..................... /Min Resp:......................./Min

Urine: Alb .... Sugar...

PHYSICAL EXAMINATION

HEAD: Hygiene...

Injury...

Surgery...

Infection ....

Any other ....

FACE: Expression...

Symmetry...

Chloasma ....

Scar...

EYES: Field of Vision...

Vision ....

Conjunctiva...

Sclera. ....

Periorbital Oedema ....

Complaints if any ....

EARS: Hygiene...

Hearing ....

Pain...

Wax...

Discharge ....

Surgery...

Complaints if any ....

NOSE: Septal Deviation ....

Discharge ....

Bleeding ....

Polyp ....

Hygiene...

Complaints if any ....

MOUTH: Lips: Colour.. Texture ....

Stomatitis:...

Hygiene:...

Halitosis: ....

Tongue: ....

Teeth: Stain...................................Symmetry..................... Caries.................................Extractions ....

Pain ....Fillings. ....

GUMS: Colour...

Bleeding ....

Gingivitis ....

Complaints if any ....

NECK: Hygiene...

Nodes ....

Glands ....

Thyroid...

Jugular Veins...

Scar...

Complaints if any ....

CHEST: Shape...

Scar. ....

LIMBS: Upper-Symmetry...

Tremors...

Nails...

Hygiene...

Infection ....

Ulnar Nerve ....

Sub.Trochlear Node...

Axilla ....

Oedema...

Lower-Symmetry...

Hygiene...

Infection ....

Nails...

Oedema...

Varicose Veins...

BACK: Hygiene...

Deformity...

Pain...

Oedema...

OBSTETRICAL EXAMINATION

BREAST: Development...

Consistency...

Symmetry...

Veins...

Areola ....

Primary...

Secondary ....

Montgomery's Tuberculosis ....

Nipples condition...

Colostrum ....

Lumps...

Axillary Nodes...

PERINEUM: Hygiene...

Discharge ....

Bleeding...

Pruritis ....

Infection...

Oedema ....

Complaints if any...

ABDOMEN

Measurements:

Fundal Height.. cms

Abdominal Girth.. cm

Gestational Age (by date)..

Inspection:

Shape...

Size ....

Hygiene...

Scars ....

Veins...

Fetal Movements...

Linea Nigra...

Striae ....

Palpation:

Fundal Palpation..

Rt. Lateral..

Lt. Lateral..

Pelvic Palpation..

Pawlick Grip..

Ausculation:

FHS..

Conclusion:

Lie..

Attitude..

Presentation..

Position..

Prest. Part: Eng/Not Engaged..

INVESTIGATION

INVESTIGATION BIOCHEMICAL										BIOPHYSICAL							
		Blood					Urine			USG							
S. No.	Date	Hb	Blood Group	HIV	VDRL	Blood Sugar	R	C	Stool	NST	BPP	FL/CRL	Placenta	Gest.Wks	LIQ	Anamoly

Any Other: ....

Treatment: Drugs..

Supportive: ....

DAILY OBSERVATION

Date	Temp	Pulse	Resp	BP	Weight	FSH	Urine output	Urine		Fundal HT	Abd. Girth	Kicks Count 4 hrly
								Albu	Sugar			

NURSING PROBLEM AND RELATED OBJECTIVE OF CARE

Actual Problem Nursing Problem..

....

....

....

....

....

Potential Problem Nursing Problem..

....

....

....

....

....

NURSING CARE PLAN

ASSESSMENT	NSG DIAGNOSIS	GOAL	PLANNING	IMPLEMENTATION

HEALTH EDUCATION

Date ....Topic..

Content

....

....

....

....

....

Teacher Signature...

ANTENATAL CARE STUDY

IDENTIFICATION DATA

Name of Mother..

Reg. No:..

Age: ....

Gravida: ....

Para:...

Diagnosis: ....

Date of Admission:...

Date of Discharge: ....

PAST MENSTRURAL HISTORY

LMP ....EDD ....Cycle..

HEALTH HISTORY

1. Past Obstetrical History..

   ....

   ....

2. Present Pregnancy History

   - I-trimester ....

     ....

     ....

   - II-trimester ....

     ....

     ....

- III-trimester...
....
....

3. Past Medical History..
....
....

4. Present Surgical History. ....
....
....

5. Past Surgical History. ....
....
....

6. Family History. ....
....
....

7. Personal History. ....
....
....

OBSTETRICAL HISTORY

S.No.	Year	Abortion	Prem	F.T.	Type of Labour and Mode of Delivery	Gender	Live or Still Birth	Remark

ANTENATAL ATTENDANCES

LMP.............................. EDD..Gestation at 1st visit.................. wk

Date	Wt	BP	FHS	Weeks	Fundal Height	Presentation	Treatments and Remarks

GENERAL EXAMINATION

Poor/Fair/Good

Height: .... cms Weight:............................ Kgs

BP: mm Hg .... Temp: ....Pulse:..................... /Min Resp:......................./Min

Urine: Alb .... Sugar..

PHYSICAL EXAMINATION

HEAD: Hygiene...

Injury...

Surgery...

Infection ....

Any other ....

FACE: Expression...

Symmetry...

Chloasma ....

Scar...

EYES: Field of Vision...

Vision ....

Conjunctiva ....

Sclera. ....

Periorbital Oedema ....

Complaints if any ....

EARS: Hygiene..

Hearing..

Pain..

Wax..

Discharge..

Surgery..

Complaints if any..

NOSE: Septal Deviation..

Discharge..

Bleeding..

Polyp..

Hygiene..

Complaints if any..

MOUTH: Lips: Colour.................................... Texture....................................

Stomatitis:..

Hygiene:..

Halitosis:..

Tongue:..

Teeth: Stain............................Symmetry..................Caries.............................Extractions.....................

Pain ....Fillings. ....

GUMS: Colour..

Bleeding..

Gingivitis..

Complaints if any..

NECK: Hygiene..

Nodes..

Glands..

Thyroid..

Jugular Veins..

Scar..

Complaints if any..

CHEST: Shape..

Scar..

LIMBS: Upper-Symmetry..

Tremors..

Nails..

Hygiene..

Infection..

Ulnar Nerve..

Sub.Trochlear Node..

Axilla..

Oedema..

Lower-Symmetry..

Hygiene..

Infection..

Nails..

Oedema..

Varicose Veins..

BACK: Hygiene..

Deformity..

Pain..

Oedema..

OBSTETRICAL EXAMINATION

BREAST: Development..

Consistency..

Symmetry..

Veins..

Areola..

Primary..

Secondary ....

Montgomery's Tuberculosis ....

Nipples condition ....

Colostrum ....

Lumps ....

Axillary Nodes ....

PERINEUM: Hygiene ....

Discharge ....

Bleeding ....

Pruritis ....

Infection ....

Oedema ....

Complaints if any ....

ABDOMEN

Measurements:

Fundal Height .... cms

Abdominal Girth .... cm

Gestational Age (by date) ....

Inspection:

Shape ....

Size ....

Hygiene ....

Scars ....

Veins ....

Fetal Movements ....

Linea Nigra ....

Striae ....

Palpation:

Fundal Palpation...

Rt. Lateral...

Lt. Lateral...

Pelvic Palpation...

Pawlick Grip...

Ausculation:

FHS...

Conclusion:

Lie...

Attitude...

Presentation...

Position...

Prest. Part: Eng/Not Engaged...

INVESTIGATION

INVESTIGATION BIOCHEMICAL										BIOPHYSICAL							
S. No.	Date	Blood					Urine		Stool	USG							
		Hb	Blood Group	HIV	VDRL	Blood Sugar	R	C		NST	BPP	FL/CRL	Placenta	Gest.Wks	LIQ	Anamoly

Any Other: ....

Treatment: Drugs...

Supportive:...

DAILY OBSERVATION

Date	Temp	Pulse	Resp	BP	Weight	FSH	Urine output	Urine		Fundal HT	Abd. Girth	Kicks Count 4 hrly
								Albu	Sugar			

NURSING PROBLEM AND RELATED OBJECTIVE OF CARE

Actual Problem Nursing Problem..

....

....

....

....

....

Potential Problem Nursing Problem..

....

....

....

....

....

NURSING CARE PLAN

ASSESSMENT	NSG DIAGNOSIS	GOAL	PLANNING	IMPLEMENTATION

HEALTH EDUCATION

Date ....Topic..

Content

....

....

....

....

....

Teacher Signature..

ANTENATAL CARE STUDY

IDENTIFICATION DATA

Name of Mother..

Reg. No:..

Age: ....

Gravida: ....

Para:..

Diagnosis: ....

Date of Admission:..

Date of Discharge: ....

PAST MENSTRUAL HISTORY

LMP .... EDD .... Cycle......................................

HEALTH HISTORY

1. Past Obstetrical History..

   ....

   ....

2. Present Pregnancy History

   - I-trimester..

     ....

     ....

   - II-trimester..

     ....

     ....

- III-trimester..

....

....

3. Past Medical History ....

....

....

4. Present Surgical History. ....

....

....

5. Past Surgical History. ....

....

....

6. Family History. ....

....

....

7. Personal History. ....

....

....

OBSTETRICAL HISTORY

S.No.	Year	Abortion	Prem	F.T.	Type of Labour and Mode of Delivery	Gender	Live or Still Birth	Remark

ANTENATAL ATTENDANCES

LMP............................ EDD...Gestation at 1st visit.................. wk

Date	Wt	BP	FHS	Weeks	Fundal Height	Presentation	Treatments and Remarks

GENERAL EXAMINATION

Poor/Fair/Good

Height: .... cms Weight:............................. Kgs

BP: mm Hg .... Temp: ....Pulse:...................... /Min Resp:......................./Min

Urine: Alb .... Sugar...

PHYSICAL EXAMINATION

HEAD: Hygiene...

Injury...

Surgery...

Infection ....

Any other ....

FACE: Expression...

Symmetry...

Chloasma ....

Scar...

EYES: Field of Vision...

Vision ....

Conjunctiva ....

Sclera. ....

Periorbital Oedema ....

Complaints if any ....

EARS: Hygiene..

Hearing..

Pain..

Wax..

Discharge..

Surgery..

Complaints if any..

NOSE: Septal Deviation..

Discharge..

Bleeding..

Polyp..

Hygiene..

Complaints if any..

MOUTH: Lips: Colour.................................... Texture....................................

Stomatitis:..

Hygiene:..

Halitosis:..

Tongue:..

Teeth: Stain..............................Symmetry...................Caries..............................Extractions......................

Pain ....Fillings. ....

GUMS: Colour..

Bleeding..

Gingivitis..

Complaints if any..

NECK: Hygiene..

Nodes..

Glands..

Thyroid..

Jugular Veins..

Scar..

Complaints if any..

CHEST: Shape..........

Scar..........

LIMBS: Upper-Symmetry..........

Tremors..........

Nails..........

Hygiene..........

Infection..........

Ulnar Nerve..........

Sub.Trochlear Node..........

Axilla..........

Oedema..........

Lower-Symmetry..........

Hygiene..........

Infection..........

Nails..........

Oedema..........

Varicose Veins..........

BACK: Hygiene..........

Deformity..........

Pain..........

Oedema..........

OBSTETRICAL EXAMINATION

BREAST: Development..........

Consistency..........

Symmetry..........

Veins..........

Areola..........

Primary..........

Secondary ....

Montgomery's Tuberculosis ....

Nipples condition..

Colostrum ....

Lumps..

Axillary Nodes..

PERINEUM: Hygiene..

Discharge ....

Bleeding..

Pruritis ....

Infection..

Oedema ....

Complaints if any..

ABDOMEN

Measurements:

Fundal Height..cms

Abdominal Girth.. cm

Gestational Age (by date)..

Inspection:

Shape..

Size ....

Hygiene..

Scars ....

Veins..

Fetal Movements..

Linea Nigra..

Striae ....

Palpation:

Fundal Palpation...

Rt. Lateral...

Lt. Lateral...

Pelvic Palpation...

Pawlick Grip...

Ausculation:

FHS...

Conclusion:

Lie...

Attitude...

Presentation...

Position...

Prest. Part: Eng/Not Engaged...

INVESTIGATION

INVESTIGATION BIOCHEMICAL											BIOPHYSICAL						
S. No.	Date	Blood					Urine		Stool	USG							
		Hb	Blood Group	HIV	VDRL	Blood Sugar	R	C		NST	BPP	FL/CRL	Placenta	Gest.Wks	LIQ	Anamoly

Any Other: ....

Treatment: Drugs...

Supportive: ....

DAILY OBSERVATION

Date	Temp	Pulse	Resp	BP	Weight	FSH	Urine output	Urine		Fundal HT	Abd. Girth	Kicks Count 4 hrly
								Albu	Sugar			

NURSING PROBLEM AND RELATED OBJECTIVE OF CARE

Actual Problem Nursing Problem..

....

....

....

....

....

Potential Problem Nursing Problem..

....

....

....

....

....

NURSING CARE PLAN

ASSESSMENT	NSG DIAGNOSIS	GOAL	PLANNING	IMPLEMENTATION

HEALTH EDUCATION

Date ....Topic..

Content

....

....

....

....

....

Teacher Signature...

ANTENATAL CARE STUDY

IDENTIFICATION DATA

Name of Mother...

Reg. No:...

Age: ....

Gravida: ....

Para:..

Diagnosis: ....

Date of Admission:..

Date of Discharge: ....

PAST MENSTRUAL HISTORY

LMP ....EDD ....Cycle..

HEALTH HISTORY

1. Past Obstetrical History...

   ....

   ....

2. Present Pregnancy History

   - I-trimester ....

     ....

     ....

   - II-trimester..

     ....

     ....

- III-trimester...

....

....

3. Past Medical History ....

....

....

4. Present Surgical History. ....

....

....

5. Past Surgical History. ....

....

....

6. Family History. ....

....

....

7. Personal History. ....

....

....

OBSTETRICAL HISTORY

S.No.	Year	Abortion	Prem	F.T.	Type of Labour and Mode of Delivery	Gender	Live or Still Birth	Remark

ANTENATAL ATTENDANCES

LMP............................ EDD...Gestation at 1st visit.................. wk

Date	Wt	BP	FHS	Weeks	Fundal Height	Presentation	Treatments and Remarks

GENERAL EXAMINATION

Poor/Fair/Good

Height: .... cms Weight:............................ Kgs

BP: mm Hg .... Temp: ....Pulse:...................... /Min Resp:........................./Min

Urine: Alb .... Sugar...

PHYSICAL EXAMINATION

HEAD: Hygiene...

Injury...

Surgery...

Infection ....

Any other ....

FACE: Expression...

Symmetry...

Chloasma ....

Scar...

EYES: Field of Vision...

Vision ....

Conjunctiva ....

Sclera. ....

Periorbital Oedema ....

Complaints if any ....

EARS: Hygiene..........

Hearing..........

Pain..........

Wax..........

Discharge..........

Surgery..........

Complaints if any..........

NOSE: Septal Deviation..........

Discharge..........

Bleeding..........

Polyp..........

Hygiene..........

Complaints if any..........

MOUTH: Lips: Colour.......... Texture..........

Stomatitis:..........

Hygiene:..........

Halitosis:..........

Tongue:..........

Teeth: Stain..........Symmetry..........Caries..........Extractions..........

Pain..........Fillings...........

GUMS: Colour..........

Bleeding..........

Gingivitis..........

Complaints if any..........

NECK: Hygiene..........

Nodes..........

Glands..........

Thyroid..........

Jugular Veins..........

Scar..........

Complaints if any..........

CHEST: Shape..

Scar. ....

LIMBS: Upper-Symmetry..

Tremors..

Nails..

Hygiene..

Infection ....

Ulnar Nerve ....

Sub.Trochlear Node..

Axilla ....

Oedema..

Lower-Symmetry..

Hygiene..

Infection ....

Nails..

Oedema..

Varicose Veins..

BACK: Hygiene..

Deformity..

Pain..

Oedema..

OBSTETRICAL EXAMINATION

BREAST: Development..

Consistency ....

Symmetry..

Veins..

Areola ....

Primary..

Secondary ....

Montgomery's Tuberculosis ....

Nipples condition ....

Colostrum ....

Lumps ....

Axillary Nodes ....

PERINEUM: Hygiene ....

Discharge ....

Bleeding ....

Pruritis ....

Infection ....

Oedema ....

Complaints if any ....

ABDOMEN

Measurements:

Fundal Height .... cms

Abdominal Girth .... cm

Gestational Age (by date) ....

Inspection:

Shape ....

Size ....

Hygiene ....

Scars ....

Veins ....

Fetal Movements ....

Linea Nigra ....

Striae ....

Palpation:

Fundal Palpation..

Rt. Lateral..

Lt. Lateral..

Pelvic Palpation..

Pawlick Grip..

Ausculation:

FHS..

Conclusion:

Lie..

Attitude..

Presentation..

Position..

Prest. Part: Eng/Not Engaged..

INVESTIGATION

INVESTIGATION BIOCHEMICAL											BIOPHYSICAL						
S. No.	Date	Blood					Urine		Stool	USG							
		Hb	Blood Group	HIV	VDRL	Blood Sugar	R	C		NST	BPP	FL/CRL	Placenta	Gest.Wks	LIQ	Anamoly

Any Other: ....

Treatment: Drugs..

Supportive: ....

DAILY OBSERVATION

Date	Temp	Pulse	Resp	BP	Weight	FSH	Urine output	Urine		Fundal HT	Abd. Girth	Kicks Count 4 hrly
								Albu	Sugar			

NURSING PROBLEM AND RELATED OBJECTIVE OF CARE

Actual Problem Nursing Problem..

....

....

....

....

....

Potential Problem Nursing Problem..

....

....

....

....

....

NURSING CARE PLAN

ASSESSMENT	NSG DIAGNOSIS	GOAL	PLANNING	IMPLEMENTATION

HEALTH EDUCATION

Date ....Topic..

Content

....

....

....

....

....

Teacher Signature...

ANTENATAL CARE STUDY

IDENTIFICATION DATA

Name of Mother..

Reg. No:..

Age: ....

Gravida: ....

Para:..

Diagnosis: ....

Date of Admission:...

Date of Discharge: ....

PAST MENSTRUAL HISTORY

LMP ....EDD ....Cycle...

HEALTH HISTORY

1. Past Obstetrical History...

   ....

   ....

2. Present Pregnancy History
   - I-trimester ....

     ....

     ....

   - II-trimester...

     ....

     ....

- III-trimester..
....
....

3. Past Medical History ....
....
....

4. Present Surgical History. ....
....
....

5. Past Surgical History. ....
....
....

6. Family History. ....
....
....

7. Personal History. ....
....
....

OBSTETRICAL HISTORY

S.No.	Year	Abortion	Prem	F.T.	Type of Labour and Mode of Delivery	Gender	Live or Still Birth	Remark

ANTENATAL ATTENDANCES

LMP............................ EDD...Gestation at 1st visit.................. wk

Date	Wt	BP	FHS	Weeks	Fundal Height	Presentation	Treatments and Remarks

GENERAL EXAMINATION

Poor/Fair/Good

Height: .... cms Weight:............................Kgs

BP: mm Hg .... Temp: ....Pulse:..................... /Min Resp:......................./Min

Urine: Alb .... Sugar...

PHYSICAL EXAMINATION

HEAD: Hygiene...

Injury...

Surgery...

Infection ....

Any other ....

FACE: Expression...

Symmetry...

Chloasma ....

Scar...

EYES: Field of Vision...

Vision ....

Conjunctiva ....

Sclera. ....

Periorbital Oedema ....

Complaints if any ....

EARS: Hygiene..........

Hearing..........

Pain..........

Wax..........

Discharge..........

Surgery..........

Complaints if any..........

NOSE: Septal Deviation..........

Discharge..........

Bleeding..........

Polyp..........

Hygiene..........

Complaints if any..........

MOUTH: Lips: Colour.......... Texture..........

Stomatitis:..........

Hygiene:..........

Halitosis:..........

Tongue:..........

Teeth: Stain..........Symmetry..........Caries..........Extractions..........

Pain..........Fillings...........

GUMS: Colour..........

Bleeding..........

Gingivitis..........

Complaints if any..........

NECK: Hygiene..........

Nodes..........

Glands..........

Thyroid..........

Jugular Veins..........

Scar..........

Complaints if any..........

CHEST: Shape..

Scar..

LIMBS: Upper-Symmetry..

Tremors..

Nails..

Hygiene..

Infection..

Ulnar Nerve..

Sub.Trochlear Node..

Axilla..

Oedema..

Lower-Symmetry..

Hygiene..

Infection..

Nails..

Oedema..

Varicose Veins..

BACK: Hygiene..

Deformity..

Pain..

Oedema..

OBSTETRICAL EXAMINATION

BREAST: Development..

Consistency..

Symmetry..

Veins..

Areola..

Primary..

Secondary ....

Montgomery's Tuberculosis ....

Nipples condition ....

Colostrum ....

Lumps ....

Axillary Nodes ....

PERINEUM: Hygiene ....

Discharge ....

Bleeding ....

Pruritis ....

Infection ....

Oedema ....

Complaints if any ....

ABDOMEN

Measurements:

Fundal Height .... cms

Abdominal Girth .... cm

Gestational Age (by date) ....

Inspection:

Shape ....

Size ....

Hygiene ....

Scars ....

Veins ....

Fetal Movements ....

Linea Nigra ....

Striae ....

Palpation:

Fundal Palpation..........

Rt. Lateral..........

Lt. Lateral..........

Pelvic Palpation..........

Pawlick Grip..........

Ausculation:

FHS..........

Conclusion:

Lie..........

Attitude..........

Presentation..........

Position..........

Prest. Part: Eng/Not Engaged..........

INVESTIGATION

INVESTIGATION BIOCHEMICAL										BIOPHYSICAL							
S. No.	Date	Blood					Urine		Stool	USG							
		Hb	Blood Group	HIV	VDRL	Blood Sugar	R	C		NST	BPP	FL/CRL	Placenta	Gest.Wks	LIQ	Anamoly

Any Other: ....

Treatment: Drugs..........

Supportive: ....

DAILY OBSERVATION

Date	Temp	Pulse	Resp	BP	Weight	FSH	Urine output	Urine		Fundal HT	Abd. Girth	Kicks Count 4 hrly
								Albu	Sugar			

NURSING PROBLEM AND RELATED OBJECTIVE OF CARE

Actual Problem Nursing Problem..

....

....

....

....

....

Potential Problem Nursing Problem..

....

....

....

....

....

NURSING CARE PLAN

ASSESSMENT	NSG DIAGNOSIS	GOAL	PLANNING	IMPLEMENTATION

HEALTH EDUCATION

Date ....Topic..

Content

....

....

....

....

....

Teacher Signature...

ANTENATAL CARE STUDY

IDENTIFICATION DATA

Name of Mother...

Reg. No:...

Age: ....

Gravida: ....

Para:...

Diagnosis: ....

Date of Admission:...

Date of Discharge: ....

PAST MENSTRUAL HISTORY

LMP ....EDD ....Cycle...

HEALTH HISTORY

1. Past Obstetrical History...

   ....

   ....

2. Present Pregnancy History

   - I-trimester...

     ....

     ....

   - II-trimester...

     ....

     ....

- III-trimester..
....
....

3. Past Medical History..
....
....

4. Present Surgical History. ....
....
....

5. Past Surgical History. ....
....
....

6. Family History. ....
....
....

7. Personal History. ....
....
....

OBSTETRICAL HISTORY

S.No.	Year	Abortion	Prem	F.T.	Type of Labour and Mode of Delivery	Gender	Live or Still Birth	Remark

ANTENATAL ATTENDANCES

LMP............................ EDD..Gestation at 1st visit.................. wk

Date	Wt	BP	FHS	Weeks	Fundal Height	Presentation	Treatments and Remarks

GENERAL EXAMINATION

Poor/Fair/Good

Height: .... cms Weight:............................ Kgs

BP: mm Hg .... Temp: ....Pulse:..................... /Min Resp:......................./Min

Urine: Alb .... Sugar...

PHYSICAL EXAMINATION

HEAD: Hygiene..

Injury..

Surgery..

Infection ....

Any other ....

FACE: Expression..

Symmetry..

Chloasma ....

Scar..

EYES: Field of Vision..

Vision ....

Conjunctiva ....

Sclera. ....

Periorbital Oedema ....

Complaints if any ....

EARS: Hygiene...

Hearing...

Pain...

Wax...

Discharge...

Surgery...

Complaints if any...

NOSE: Septal Deviation...

Discharge...

Bleeding...

Polyp...

Hygiene...

Complaints if any...

MOUTH: Lips: Colour.................................... Texture..

Stomatitis:...

Hygiene:...

Halitosis:...

Tongue:...

Teeth: Stain................................Symmetry.................. Caries.............................Extractions.....................

Pain ....Fillings. ....

GUMS: Colour...

Bleeding...

Gingivitis...

Complaints if any...

NECK: Hygiene...

Nodes...

Glands...

Thyroid...

Jugular Veins...

Scar...

Complaints if any...

CHEST: Shape..........

Scar..........

LIMBS: Upper-Symmetry..........

Tremors..........

Nails..........

Hygiene..........

Infection..........

Ulnar Nerve..........

Sub.Trochlear Node..........

Axilla..........

Oedema..........

Lower-Symmetry..........

Hygiene..........

Infection..........

Nails..........

Oedema..........

Varicose Veins..........

BACK: Hygiene..........

Deformity..........

Pain..........

Oedema..........

OBSTETRICAL EXAMINATION

BREAST: Development..........

Consistency..........

Symmetry..........

Veins..........

Areola..........

Primary..........

Secondary ....

Montgomery's Tuberculosis ....

Nipples condition..

Colostrum ....

Lumps...

Axillary Nodes...

PERINEUM: Hygiene...

Discharge ....

Bleeding...

Pruritis ....

Infection...

Oedema ....

Complaints if any...

ABDOMEN

Measurements:

Fundal Height.. cms

Abdominal Girth.. cm

Gestational Age (by date)..

Inspection:

Shape...

Size ....

Hygiene..

Scars ....

Veins..

Fetal Movements...

Linea Nigra...

Striae ....

Palpation:

Fundal Palpation..........

Rt. Lateral..........

Lt. Lateral..........

Pelvic Palpation..........

Pawlick Grip..........

Ausculation:

FHS..........

Conclusion:

Lie..........

Attitude..........

Presentation..........

Position..........

Prest. Part: Eng/Not Engaged..........

INVESTIGATION

INVESTIGATION BIOCHEMICAL										BIOPHYSICAL						
S. No.	Date	Blood					Urine		Stool	USG						
		Hb	Blood Group	HIV	VDRL	Blood Sugar	R	C		NST	BPP	FL/CRL	Placenta	Gest.Wks	LIQ	Anamoly

Any Other: ....

Treatment: Drugs..........

Supportive: ....

DAILY OBSERVATION

Date	Temp	Pulse	Resp	BP	Weight	FSH	Urine output	Urine		Fundal HT	Abd. Girth	Kicks Count 4 hrly
								Albu	Sugar			

NURSING PROBLEM AND RELATED OBJECTIVE OF CARE

Actual Problem Nursing Problem...

....

....

....

....

....

Potential Problem Nursing Problem...

....

....

....

....

....

NURSING CARE PLAN

ASSESSMENT	NSG DIAGNOSIS	GOAL	PLANNING	IMPLEMENTATION

HEALTH EDUCATION

Date ....Topic...

Content

....

....

....

....

....

Teacher Signature..

ANTENATAL CARE STUDY

IDENTIFICATION DATA

Name of Mother...

Reg. No:..

Age: ....

Gravida: ....

Para:..

Diagnosis: ....

Date of Admission:...

Date of Discharge: ....

PAST MENSTRUAL HISTORY

LMP .... EDD .... Cycle..

HEALTH HISTORY

1. Past Obstetrical History...

   ....

   ....

2. Present Pregnancy History

   - I-trimester ....

     ....

     ....

   - II-trimester ....

     ....

     ....

- III-trimester..

3. Past Medical History..

4. Present Surgical History..

5. Past Surgical History..

6. Family History..

7. Personal History..

OBSTETRICAL HISTORY

S.No.	Year	Abortion	Prem	F.T.	Type of Labour and Mode of Delivery	Gender	Live or Still Birth	Remark

ANTENATAL ATTENDANCES

LMP............................. EDD..Gestation at 1st visit................... wk

Date	Wt	BP	FHS	Weeks	Fundal Height	Presentation	Treatments and Remarks

GENERAL EXAMINATION

Poor/Fair/Good

Height: .... cms Weight:............................ Kgs

BP: mm Hg .... Temp: ....Pulse:..................... /Min Resp:......................./Min

Urine: Alb .... Sugar..

PHYSICAL EXAMINATION

HEAD: Hygiene...

Injury...

Surgery...

Infection ....

Any other ....

FACE: Expression...

Symmetry...

Chloasma ....

Scar...

EYES: Field of Vision...

Vision ....

Conjunctiva...

Sclera. ....

Periorbital Oedema ....

Complaints if any ....

EARS: Hygiene..

Hearing..

Pain..

Wax..

Discharge..

Surgery..

Complaints if any..

NOSE: Septal Deviation..

Discharge..

Bleeding..

Polyp..

Hygiene..

Complaints if any..

MOUTH: Lips: Colour.................................... Texture..

Stomatitis:..

Hygiene:..

Halitosis:..

Tongue:..

Teeth: Stain.................................Symmetry...................... Caries................................Extractions.......................

Pain ....Fillings. ....

GUMS: Colour..

Bleeding..

Gingivitis..

Complaints if any..

NECK: Hygiene..

Nodes..

Glands..

Thyroid..

Jugular Veins..

Scar..

Complaints if any..

CHEST: Shape..

Scar. ....

LIMBS: Upper-Symmetry..

Tremors..

Nails..

Hygiene..

Infection ....

Ulnar Nerve ....

Sub.Trochlear Node..

Axilla ....

Oedema..

Lower-Symmetry..

Hygiene..

Infection ....

Nails..

Oedema..

Varicose Veins..

BACK: Hygiene..

Deformity..

Pain..

Oedema..

OBSTETRICAL EXAMINATION

BREAST: Development..

Consistency ....

Symmetry..

Veins..

Areola ....

Primary..

Secondary ....

Montgomery's Tuberculosis ....

Nipples condition ....

Colostrum ....

Lumps ....

Axillary Nodes ....

PERINEUM: Hygiene ....

Discharge ....

Bleeding ....

Pruritis ....

Infection ....

Oedema ....

Complaints if any ....

ABDOMEN

Measurements:

Fundal Height .... cms

Abdominal Girth .... cm

Gestational Age (by date) ....

Inspection:

Shape ....

Size ....

Hygiene ....

Scars ....

Veins ....

Fetal Movements ....

Linea Nigra ....

Striae ....

Palpation:

Fundal Palpation..........

Rt. Lateral..........

Lt. Lateral..........

Pelvic Palpation..........

Pawlick Grip..........

Ausculation:

FHS..........

Conclusion:

Lie..........

Attitude..........

Presentation..........

Position..........

Prest. Part: Eng/Not Engaged..........

INVESTIGATION

INVESTIGATION BIOCHEMICAL											BIOPHYSICAL						
S. No.	Date	Blood					Urine		Stool	USG							
		Hb	Blood Group	HIV	VDRL	Blood Sugar	R	C		NST	BPP	FL/CRL	Placenta	Gest.Wks	LIQ	Anamoly

Any Other: ....

Treatment: Drugs..........

Supportive: ....

DAILY OBSERVATION

Date	Temp	Pulse	Resp	BP	Weight	FSH	Urine output	Urine		Fundal HT	Abd. Girth	Kicks Count 4 hrly
								Albu	Sugar			

NURSING PROBLEM AND RELATED OBJECTIVE OF CARE

Actual Problem Nursing Problem..

....

....

....

....

....

Potential Problem Nursing Problem...

....

....

....

....

....

NURSING CARE PLAN

ASSESSMENT	NSG DIAGNOSIS	GOAL	PLANNING	IMPLEMENTATION

HEALTH EDUCATION

Date ....Topic..

Content

....

....

....

....

....

Teacher Signature...

ANTENATAL CARE STUDY

IDENTIFICATION DATA

Name of Mother..

Reg. No:..

Age: ....

Gravida: ....

Para:..

Diagnosis: ....

Date of Admission:..

Date of Discharge: ....

PAST MENSTRUAL HISTORY

LMP .... EDD .... Cycle...

HEALTH HISTORY

1. Past Obstetrical History..

   ....

   ....

2. Present Pregnancy History

   - I-trimester ....

     ....

     ....

   - II-trimester..

     ....

     ....

- III-trimester..

....

....

3. Past Medical History..

....

....

4. Present Surgical History...

....

....

5. Past Surgical History...

....

....

6. Family History...

....

....

7. Personal History...

....

....

OBSTETRICAL HISTORY

S.No.	Year	Abortion	Prem	F.T.	Type of Labour and Mode of Delivery	Gender	Live or Still Birth	Remark

ANTENATAL ATTENDANCES

LMP............................ EDD...Gestation at 1st visit.................. wk

Date	Wt	BP	FHS	Weeks	Fundal Height	Presentation	Treatments and Remarks

GENERAL EXAMINATION

Poor/Fair/Good

Height: .... cms Weight:............................Kgs

BP: mm Hg .... Temp: ....Pulse:..................... /Min Resp:......................./Min

Urine: Alb .... Sugar..

PHYSICAL EXAMINATION

HEAD: Hygiene..

Injury..

Surgery..

Infection ....

Any other ....

FACE: Expression..

Symmetry..

Chloasma ....

Scar..

EYES: Field of Vision..

Vision ....

Conjunctiva ....

Sclera. ....

Periorbital Oedema ....

Complaints if any ....

EARS: Hygiene...

Hearing...

Pain...

Wax...

Discharge...

Surgery...

Complaints if any...

NOSE: Septal Deviation...

Discharge...

Bleeding...

Polyp...

Hygiene...

Complaints if any...

MOUTH: Lips: Colour.................................... Texture....................................

Stomatitis:...

Hygiene:...

Halitosis:...

Tongue:...

Teeth: Stain................................Symmetry...................Caries................................Extractions......................

Pain ....Fillings. ....

GUMS: Colour...

Bleeding...

Gingivitis...

Complaints if any...

NECK: Hygiene...

Nodes...

Glands...

Thyroid...

Jugular Veins...

Scar...

Complaints if any...

CHEST: Shape...

Scar. ....

LIMBS: Upper-Symmetry...

Tremors...

Nails...

Hygiene...

Infection ....

Ulnar Nerve ....

Sub.Trochlear Node...

Axilla ....

Oedema...

Lower-Symmetry...

Hygiene...

Infection ....

Nails...

Oedema...

Varicose Veins...

BACK: Hygiene...

Deformity...

Pain...

Oedema...

OBSTETRICAL EXAMINATION

BREAST: Development...

Consistency ....

Symmetry...

Veins...

Areola ....

Primary...

Secondary ....

Montgomery's Tuberculosis ....

Nipples condition ....

Colostrum ....

Lumps ....

Axillary Nodes ....

PERINEUM: Hygiene ....

Discharge ....

Bleeding ....

Pruritis ....

Infection ....

Oedema ....

Complaints if any ....

ABDOMEN

Measurements:

Fundal Height .... cms

Abdominal Girth .... cm

Gestational Age (by date) ....

Inspection:

Shape ....

Size ....

Hygiene ....

Scars ....

Veins ....

Fetal Movements ....

Linea Nigra ....

Striae ....

Palpation:

Fundal Palpation..........

Rt. Lateral..........

Lt. Lateral..........

Pelvic Palpation..........

Pawlick Grip..........

Ausculation:

FHS..........

Conclusion:

Lie..........

Attitude..........

Presentation..........

Position..........

Prest. Part: Eng/Not Engaged..........

INVESTIGATION

INVESTIGATION BIOCHEMICAL										BIOPHYSICAL						
S. No.	Date	Blood					Urine		Stool	USG						
		Hb	Blood Group	HIV	VDRL	Blood Sugar	R	C		NST	BPP	FL/CRL	Placenta	Gest.Wks	LIQ	Anamoly

Any Other: ....

Treatment: Drugs..........

Supportive: ....

DAILY OBSERVATION

Date	Temp	Pulse	Resp	BP	Weight	FSH	Urine output	Urine		Fundal HT	Abd. Girth	Kicks Count 4 hrly
								Albu	Sugar			

NURSING PROBLEM AND RELATED OBJECTIVE OF CARE

Actual Problem Nursing Problem..

....

....

....

....

....

Potential Problem Nursing Problem..

....

....

....

....

....

NURSING CARE PLAN

ASSESSMENT	NSG DIAGNOSIS	GOAL	PLANNING	IMPLEMENTATION

HEALTH EDUCATION

Date ....Topic...

Content

....

....

....

....

....

Teacher Signature...

ANTENATAL CARE STUDY

IDENTIFICATION DATA

Name of Mother...

Reg. No:...

Age: ....

Gravida: ....

Para:...

Diagnosis: ....

Date of Admission:...

Date of Discharge: ....

PAST MENSTRUAL HISTORY

LMP .... EDD .... Cycle ....

HEALTH HISTORY

1. Past Obstetrical History...

   ....

   ....

2. Present Pregnancy History

   - I-trimester ....

     ....

     ....

   - II-trimester ....

     ....

     ....

- III-trimester..
  ....
  ....

3. Past Medical History..
   ....
   ....

4. Present Surgical History. ....
   ....
   ....

5. Past Surgical History. ....
   ....
   ....

6. Family History. ....
   ....
   ....

7. Personal History. ....
   ....
   ....

OBSTETRICAL HISTORY

S.No.	Year	Abortion	Prem	F.T.	Type of Labour and Mode of Delivery	Gender	Live or Still Birth	Remark

ANTENATAL ATTENDANCES

LMP.............................. EDD..Gestation at 1st visit.................. wk

Date	Wt	BP	FHS	Weeks	Fundal Height	Presentation	Treatments and Remarks

GENERAL EXAMINATION

Poor/Fair/Good

Height: .... cms Weight:............................Kgs

BP: mm Hg .... Temp: ....Pulse:..................... /Min Resp:.......................</Min

Urine: Alb .... Sugar...

PHYSICAL EXAMINATION

HEAD: Hygiene..

Injury..

Surgery..

Infection ....

Any other ....

FACE: Expression..

Symmetry..

Chloasma ....

Scar..

EYES: Field of Vision..

Vision ....

Conjunctiva ....

Sclera. ....

Periorbital Oedema ....

Complaints if any ....

EARS: Hygiene..

Hearing..

Pain..

Wax..

Discharge..

Surgery..

Complaints if any..

NOSE: Septal Deviation..

Discharge..

Bleeding..

Polyp..

Hygiene..

Complaints if any..

MOUTH: Lips: Colour........................ Texture........................

Stomatitis:..

Hygiene:..

Halitosis:..

Tongue:..

Teeth: Stain....................Symmetry....................Caries....................Extractions....................

Pain ....Fillings. ....

GUMS: Colour..

Bleeding..

Gingivitis..

Complaints if any..

NECK: Hygiene..

Nodes..

Glands..

Thyroid..

Jugular Veins..

Scar..

Complaints if any..

CHEST: Shape..

Scar..

LIMBS: Upper-Symmetry..

Tremors..

Nails..

Hygiene..

Infection..

Ulnar Nerve..

Sub.Trochlear Node..

Axilla..

Oedema..

Lower-Symmetry..

Hygiene..

Infection..

Nails..

Oedema..

Varicose Veins..

BACK: Hygiene..

Deformity..

Pain..

Oedema..

OBSTETRICAL EXAMINATION

BREAST: Development..

Consistency..

Symmetry..

Veins..

Areola..

Primary..

Secondary ....

Montgomery's Tuberculosis ....

Nipples condition ....

Colostrum ....

Lumps ....

Axillary Nodes ....

PERINEUM: Hygiene ....

Discharge ....

Bleeding ....

Pruritis ....

Infection ....

Oedema ....

Complaints if any ....

ABDOMEN

Measurements:

Fundal Height .... cms

Abdominal Girth .... cm

Gestational Age (by date) ....

Inspection:

Shape ....

Size ....

Hygiene ....

Scars ....

Veins ....

Fetal Movements ....

Linea Nigra ....

Striae ....

Palpation:

Fundal Palpation..........

Rt. Lateral..........

Lt. Lateral..........

Pelvic Palpation..........

Pawlick Grip..........

Ausculation:

FHS..........

Conclusion:

Lie..........

Attitude..........

Presentation..........

Position..........

Prest. Part: Eng/Not Engaged..........

INVESTIGATION

INVESTIGATION BIOCHEMICAL											BIOPHYSICAL						
		Blood					Urine			USG							
S. No.	Date	Hb	Blood Group	HIV	VDRL	Blood Sugar	R	C	Stool	NST	BPP	FL/CRL	Placenta	Gest.Wks	LIQ	Anamoly

Any Other: ....

Treatment: Drugs..........

Supportive: ....

DAILY OBSERVATION

Date	Temp	Pulse	Resp	BP	Weight	FSH	Urine output	Urine		Fundal HT	Abd. Girth	Kicks Count 4 hrly
								Albu	Sugar			

NURSING PROBLEM AND RELATED OBJECTIVE OF CARE

Actual Problem Nursing Problem..

....

....

....

....

....

Potential Problem Nursing Problem..

....

....

....

....

....

NURSING CARE PLAN

ASSESSMENT	NSG DIAGNOSIS	GOAL	PLANNING	IMPLEMENTATION

HEALTH EDUCATION

Date ....Topic...

Content

....

....

....

....

....

Teacher Signature...

ANTENATAL CARE STUDY

IDENTIFICATION DATA

Name of Mother..

Reg. No:...

Age: ....

Gravida: ....

Para:..

Diagnosis: ....

Date of Admission:...

Date of Discharge: ....

PAST MENSTRURAL HISTORY

LMP ....EDD ....Cycle...

HEALTH HISTORY

1. Past Obstetrical History..

   ....

   ....

2. Present Pregnancy History
   - I-trimester ....

     ....

     ....

   - II-trimester..

     ....

     ....

- III-trimester..

....

....

3. Past Medical History..

....

....

4. Present Surgical History. ....

....

....

5. Past Surgical History. ....

....

....

6. Family History. ....

....

....

7. Personal History. ....

....

....

OBSTETRICAL HISTORY

S.No.	Year	Abortion	Prem	F.T.	Type of Labour and Mode of Delivery	Gender	Live or Still Birth	Remark

ANTENATAL ATTENDANCES

LMP............................ EDD...Gestation at 1st visit.................. wk

Date	Wt	BP	FHS	Weeks	Fundal Height	Presentation	Treatments and Remarks

GENERAL EXAMINATION

Poor/Fair/Good

Height: .... cms Weight:............................Kgs

BP: mm Hg .... Temp: ....Pulse:...................... /Min Resp:........................./Min

Urine: Alb .... Sugar...

PHYSICAL EXAMINATION

HEAD: Hygiene...

Injury...

Surgery...

Infection ....

Any other ....

FACE: Expression...

Symmetry...

Chloasma ....

Scar...

EYES: Field of Vision...

Vision ....

Conjunctiva ....

Sclera. ....

Periorbital Oedema ....

Complaints if any ....

EARS: Hygiene..

Hearing ....

Pain..

Wax..

Discharge ....

Surgery..

Complaints if any ....

NOSE: Septal Deviation ....

Discharge ....

Bleeding ....

Polyp..

Hygiene..

Complaints if any ....

MOUTH: Lips: Colour.. Texture ....

Stomatitis:..

Hygiene:..

Halitosis: ....

Tongue: ....

Teeth: Stain.............................Symmetry....................Caries................................Extractions ....

Pain ....Fillings. ....

GUMS: Colour..

Bleeding ....

Gingivitis ....

Complaints if any ....

NECK: Hygiene..

Nodes ....

Glands ....

Thyroid..

Jugular Veins..

Scar..

Complaints if any ....

CHEST: Shape...

Scar. ....

LIMBS: Upper-Symmetry...

Tremors...

Nails...

Hygiene...

Infection ....

Ulnar Nerve ....

Sub.Trochlear Node...

Axilla ....

Oedema...

Lower-Symmetry...

Hygiene...

Infection ....

Nails...

Oedema...

Varicose Veins...

BACK: Hygiene...

Deformity...

Pain...

Oedema...

OBSTETRICAL EXAMINATION

BREAST: Development...

Consistency ....

Symmetry...

Veins...

Areola ....

Primary...

Secondary ....

Montgomery's Tuberculosis ....

Nipples condition ....

Colostrum ....

Lumps ....

Axillary Nodes ....

PERINEUM: Hygiene ....

Discharge ....

Bleeding ....

Pruritis ....

Infection ....

Oedema ....

Complaints if any ....

ABDOMEN

Measurements:

Fundal Height .... cms

Abdominal Girth .... cm

Gestational Age (by date) ....

Inspection:

Shape ....

Size ....

Hygiene ....

Scars ....

Veins ....

Fetal Movements ....

Linea Nigra ....

Striae ....

Palpation:

Fundal Palpation..........

Rt. Lateral..........

Lt. Lateral..........

Pelvic Palpation..........

Pawlick Grip..........

Ausculation:

FHS..........

Conclusion:

Lie..........

Attitude..........

Presentation..........

Position..........

Prest. Part: Eng/Not Engaged..........

INVESTIGATION

INVESTIGATION BIOCHEMICAL										BIOPHYSICAL							
S. No.	Date	Blood					Urine		Stool	USG							
		Hb	Blood Group	HIV	VDRL	Blood Sugar	R	C		NST	BPP	FL/CRL	Placenta	Gest.Wks	LIQ	Anamoly

Any Other: ....

Treatment: Drugs..........

Supportive: ....

DAILY OBSERVATION

Date	Temp	Pulse	Resp	BP	Weight	FSH	Urine output	Urine		Fundal HT	Abd. Girth	Kicks Count 4 hrly
								Albu	Sugar			

NURSING PROBLEM AND RELATED OBJECTIVE OF CARE

Actual Problem Nursing Problem..

....

....

....

....

....

Potential Problem Nursing Problem..

....

....

....

....

....

NURSING CARE PLAN

ASSESSMENT	NSG DIAGNOSIS	GOAL	PLANNING	IMPLEMENTATION

HEALTH EDUCATION

Date ....Topic...

Content

....

....

....

....

....

Teacher Signature...

ANTENATAL CARE STUDY

IDENTIFICATION DATA

Name of Mother...

Reg. No:...

Age: ....

Gravida: ....

Para:..

Diagnosis: ....

Date of Admission:...

Date of Discharge: ....

PAST MENSTRUAL HISTORY

LMP ....EDD ....Cycle...

HEALTH HISTORY

1. Past Obstetrical History...

   ....

   ....

2. Present Pregnancy History

   - I-trimester ....

     ....

     ....

   - II-trimester...

     ....

     ....

- III-trimester..

3. Past Medical History..

4. Present Surgical History..

5. Past Surgical History..

6. Family History..

7. Personal History..

OBSTETRICAL HISTORY

S.No.	Year	Abortion	Prem	F.T.	Type of Labour and Mode of Delivery	Gender	Live or Still Birth	Remark

ANTENATAL ATTENDANCES							
LMP............................ EDD..Gestation at 1st visit.................. wk							
Date	Wt	BP	FHS	Weeks	Fundal Height	Presentation	Treatments and Remarks

GENERAL EXAMINATION

Poor/Fair/Good

Height: .... cms Weight:............................ Kgs

BP: mm Hg .... Temp: ....Pulse:..................... /Min Resp:......................./Min

Urine: Alb .... Sugar...

PHYSICAL EXAMINATION

HEAD: Hygiene...

Injury...

Surgery...

Infection ....

Any other ....

FACE: Expression...

Symmetry...

Chloasma ....

Scar...

EYES: Field of Vision...

Vision ....

Conjunctiva ....

Sclera. ....

Periorbital Oedema ....

Complaints if any ....

EARS: Hygiene..

Hearing ....

Pain..

Wax..

Discharge ....

Surgery..

Complaints if any ....

NOSE: Septal Deviation ....

Discharge ....

Bleeding ....

Polyp ....

Hygiene..

Complaints if any ....

MOUTH: Lips: Colour.. Texture ....

Stomatitis:..

Hygiene:..

Halitosis: ....

Tongue: ....

Teeth: Stain..................................Symmetry..................... Caries..................................Extractions ....

Pain ....Fillings. ....

GUMS: Colour..

Bleeding ....

Gingivitis ....

Complaints if any ....

NECK: Hygiene..

Nodes ....

Glands ....

Thyroid..

Jugular Veins..

Scar..

Complaints if any ....

CHEST: Shape..

Scar. ....

LIMBS: Upper-Symmetry..

Tremors..

Nails..

Hygiene..

Infection ....

Ulnar Nerve ....

Sub.Trochlear Node..

Axilla ....

Oedema..

Lower-Symmetry..

Hygiene..

Infection ....

Nails..

Oedema..

Varicose Veins..

BACK: Hygiene..

Deformity..

Pain..

Oedema..

OBSTETRICAL EXAMINATION

BREAST: Development..

Consistency ....

Symmetry..

Veins..

Areola ....

Primary..

Secondary ....

Montgomery's Tuberculosis ....

Nipples condition ....

Colostrum ....

Lumps ....

Axillary Nodes ....

PERINEUM: Hygiene ....

Discharge ....

Bleeding ....

Pruritis ....

Infection ....

Oedema ....

Complaints if any ....

ABDOMEN

Measurements:

Fundal Height .... cms

Abdominal Girth .... cm

Gestational Age (by date) ....

Inspection:

Shape ....

Size ....

Hygiene ....

Scars ....

Veins ....

Fetal Movements ....

Linea Nigra ....

Striae ....

Palpation:

Fundal Palpation..........

Rt. Lateral..........

Lt. Lateral..........

Pelvic Palpation..........

Pawlick Grip..........

Ausculation:

FHS..........

Conclusion:

Lie..........

Attitude..........

Presentation..........

Position..........

Prest. Part: Eng/Not Engaged..........

INVESTIGATION

INVESTIGATION BIOCHEMICAL											BIOPHYSICAL					
		Blood					Urine			USG						
S. No.	Date	Hb	Blood Group	HIV	VDRL	Blood Sugar	R	C	Stool	NST	BPP	FL/CRL	Placenta	Gest.Wks	LIQ	Anamoly

Any Other: ....

Treatment: Drugs..........

Supportive: ....

DAILY OBSERVATION

Date	Temp	Pulse	Resp	BP	Weight	FSH	Urine output	Urine		Fundal HT	Abd. Girth	Kicks Count 4 hrly
								Albu	Sugar			

NURSING PROBLEM AND RELATED OBJECTIVE OF CARE

Actual Problem Nursing Problem..

....

....

....

....

....

Potential Problem Nursing Problem..

....

....

....

....

....

NURSING CARE PLAN

ASSESSMENT	NSG DIAGNOSIS	GOAL	PLANNING	IMPLEMENTATION

HEALTH EDUCATION

Date ....Topic...

Content

....

....

....

....

....

Teacher Signature..

ANTENATAL CARE STUDY

IDENTIFICATION DATA

Name of Mother...

Reg. No:...

Age: ....

Gravida: ....

Para:...

Diagnosis: ....

Date of Admission:...

Date of Discharge: ....

PAST MENSTRUAL HISTORY

LMP ....EDD ....Cycle...

HEALTH HISTORY

1. Past Obstetrical History...

   ....

   ....

2. Present Pregnancy History

   - I-trimester ....

     ....

     ....

   - II-trimester...

     ....

     ....

- III-trimester...

....

....

3. Past Medical History ....

....

....

4. Present Surgical History. ....

....

....

5. Past Surgical History. ....

....

....

6. Family History. ....

....

....

7. Personal History. ....

....

....

OBSTETRICAL HISTORY

S.No.	Year	Abortion	Prem	F.T.	Type of Labour and Mode of Delivery	Gender	Live or Still Birth	Remark

ANTENATAL ATTENDANCES

LMP............................ EDD..Gestation at 1st visit.................. wk

Date	Wt	BP	FHS	Weeks	Fundal Height	Presentation	Treatments and Remarks

GENERAL EXAMINATION

Poor/Fair/Good

Height: .... cms Weight:............................Kgs

BP: mm Hg .... Temp: ....Pulse:..................... /Min Resp:......................./Min

Urine: Alb .... Sugar...

PHYSICAL EXAMINATION

HEAD: Hygiene...

Injury...

Surgery...

Infection ....

Any other ....

FACE: Expression...

Symmetry...

Chloasma ....

Scar...

EYES: Field of Vision...

Vision ....

Conjunctiva ....

Sclera. ....

Periorbital Oedema ....

Complaints if any ....

EARS: Hygiene..

Hearing..

Pain..

Wax..

Discharge..

Surgery..

Complaints if any..

NOSE: Septal Deviation..

Discharge..

Bleeding..

Polyp..

Hygiene..

Complaints if any..

MOUTH: Lips: Colour.............................. Texture..............................

Stomatitis:..

Hygiene:..

Halitosis:..

Tongue:..

Teeth: Stain..............................Symmetry..................Caries..............................Extractions......................

Pain ....Fillings. ....

GUMS: Colour..

Bleeding..

Gingivitis..

Complaints if any..

NECK: Hygiene..

Nodes..

Glands..

Thyroid..

Jugular Veins..

Scar..

Complaints if any..

CHEST: Shape...

Scar. ....

LIMBS: Upper-Symmetry...

Tremors...

Nails...

Hygiene...

Infection ....

Ulnar Nerve ....

Sub.Trochlear Node...

Axilla ....

Oedema...

Lower-Symmetry...

Hygiene...

Infection ....

Nails...

Oedema...

Varicose Veins...

BACK: Hygiene...

Deformity...

Pain...

Oedema...

OBSTETRICAL EXAMINATION

BREAST: Development...

Consistency ....

Symmetry...

Veins...

Areola ....

Primary...

Secondary ....

Montgomery's Tuberculosis ....

Nipples condition ....

Colostrum ....

Lumps ....

Axillary Nodes ....

PERINEUM: Hygiene ....

Discharge ....

Bleeding ....

Pruritis ....

Infection ....

Oedema ....

Complaints if any ....

ABDOMEN

Measurements:

Fundal Height .... cms

Abdominal Girth .... cm

Gestational Age (by date) ....

Inspection:

Shape ....

Size ....

Hygiene ....

Scars ....

Veins ....

Fetal Movements ....

Linea Nigra ....

Striae ....

Palpation:

Fundal Palpation..

Rt. Lateral..

Lt. Lateral..

Pelvic Palpation..

Pawlick Grip..

Ausculation:

FHS..

Conclusion:

Lie..

Attitude..

Presentation..

Position..

Prest. Part: Eng/Not Engaged..

INVESTIGATION

INVESTIGATION BIOCHEMICAL										BIOPHYSICAL							
		Blood					Urine			USG							
S. No.	Date	Hb	Blood Group	HIV	VDRL	Blood Sugar	R	C	Stool	NST	BPP	FL/CRL	Placenta	Gest.Wks	LIQ	Anamoly

Any Other: ....

Treatment: Drugs..

Supportive: ....

DAILY OBSERVATION

Date	Temp	Pulse	Resp	BP	Weight	FSH	Urine output	Urine		Fundal HT	Abd. Girth	Kicks Count 4 hrly
								Albu	Sugar			

NURSING PROBLEM AND RELATED OBJECTIVE OF CARE

Actual Problem Nursing Problem..

....

....

....

....

....

Potential Problem Nursing Problem..

....

....

....

....

....

NURSING CARE PLAN

ASSESSMENT	NSG DIAGNOSIS	GOAL	PLANNING	IMPLEMENTATION

HEALTH EDUCATION

Date ....Topic...

Content

....

....

....

....

....

Teacher Signature..

ANTENATAL CARE STUDY

IDENTIFICATION DATA

Name of Mother............

Reg. No:............

Age: ....

Gravida: ....

Para:............

Diagnosis: ....

Date of Admission:............

Date of Discharge: ....

PAST MENSTRUAL HISTORY

LMP .... EDD .... Cycle............

HEALTH HISTORY

1. Past Obstetrical History............

....

....

2. Present Pregnancy History

- I-trimester ....

  ....

  ....

- II-trimester............

  ....

  ....

- III-trimester..

3. Past Medical History..

4. Present Surgical History...

5. Past Surgical History..

6. Family History...

7. Personal History..

OBSTETRICAL HISTORY

S.No.	Year	Abortion	Prem	F.T.	Type of Labour and Mode of Delivery	Gender	Live or Still Birth	Remark

ANTENATAL ATTENDANCES

LMP............................ EDD...Gestation at 1st visit.................. wk

Date	Wt	BP	FHS	Weeks	Fundal Height	Presentation	Treatments and Remarks

GENERAL EXAMINATION

Poor/Fair/Good

Height: .... cms Weight:............................Kgs

BP: mm Hg .... Temp: ....Pulse:..................... /Min Resp:......................../Min

Urine: Alb .... Sugar...

PHYSICAL EXAMINATION

HEAD: Hygiene...

Injury...

Surgery...

Infection ....

Any other ....

FACE: Expression...

Symmetry...

Chloasma ....

Scar...

EYES: Field of Vision...

Vision ....

Conjunctiva ....

Sclera. ....

Periorbital Oedema ....

Complaints if any ....

EARS: Hygiene...

Hearing ....

Pain...

Wax...

Discharge ....

Surgery...

Complaints if any ....

NOSE: Septal Deviation ....

Discharge ....

Bleeding ....

Polyp ....

Hygiene...

Complaints if any ....

MOUTH: Lips: Colour....................................... Texture ....

Stomatitis:...

Hygiene:...

Halitosis: ....

Tongue:...

Teeth: Stain..................................Symmetry....................Caries.................................Extractions ....

Pain ....Fillings. ....

GUMS: Colour...

Bleeding ....

Gingivitis ....

Complaints if any ....

NECK: Hygiene...

Nodes ....

Glands ....

Thyroid...

Jugular Veins...

Scar...

Complaints if any ....

CHEST: Shape...

Scar. ....

LIMBS: Upper-Symmetry...

Tremors...

Nails...

Hygiene...

Infection ....

Ulnar Nerve ....

Sub.Trochlear Node...

Axilla ....

Oedema...

Lower-Symmetry...

Hygiene...

Infection ....

Nails...

Oedema...

Varicose Veins...

BACK: Hygiene...

Deformity...

Pain...

Oedema...

OBSTETRICAL EXAMINATION

BREAST: Development...

Consistency ....

Symmetry...

Veins...

Areola ....

Primary...

Secondary ....

Montgomery's Tuberculosis ....

Nipples condition ....

Colostrum ....

Lumps ....

Axillary Nodes ....

PERINEUM: Hygiene ....

Discharge ....

Bleeding ....

Pruritis ....

Infection ....

Oedema ....

Complaints if any ....

ABDOMEN

Measurements:

Fundal Height .... cms

Abdominal Girth .... cm

Gestational Age (by date) ....

Inspection:

Shape ....

Size ....

Hygiene ....

Scars ....

Veins ....

Fetal Movements ....

Linea Nigra ....

Striae ....

Palpation:

Fundal Palpation...

Rt. Lateral...

Lt. Lateral...

Pelvic Palpation...

Pawlick Grip...

Ausculation:

FHS...

Conclusion:

Lie...

Attitude...

Presentation...

Position...

Prest. Part: Eng/Not Engaged...

INVESTIGATION

INVESTIGATION BIOCHEMICAL										BIOPHYSICAL							
		Blood					Urine			USG							
S. No.	Date	Hb	Blood Group	HIV	VDRL	Blood Sugar	R	C	Stool	NST	BPP	FL/CRL	Placenta	Gest.Wks	LIQ	Anamoly

Any Other: ....

Treatment: Drugs...

Supportive: ....

DAILY OBSERVATION

Date	Temp	Pulse	Resp	BP	Weight	FSH	Urine output	Urine		Fundal HT	Abd. Girth	Kicks Count 4 hrly
								Albu	Sugar			

NURSING PROBLEM AND RELATED OBJECTIVE OF CARE

Actual Problem Nursing Problem..

....

....

....

....

....

Potential Problem Nursing Problem..

....

....

....

....

....

NURSING CARE PLAN

ASSESSMENT	NSG DIAGNOSIS	GOAL	PLANNING	IMPLEMENTATION

HEALTH EDUCATION

Date .... Topic..

Content

....

....

....

....

....

Teacher Signature...

ANTENATAL CARE STUDY

IDENTIFICATION DATA

Name of Mother..

Reg. No:...

Age: ....

Gravida: ....

Para:...

Diagnosis: ....

Date of Admission:..

Date of Discharge: ....

PAST MENSTRUAL HISTORY

LMP .... EDD .... Cycle ....

HEALTH HISTORY

1. Past Obstetrical History..

   ....

   ....

2. Present Pregnancy History

   - I-trimester ....

     ....

     ....

   - II-trimester ....

     ....

     ....

- III-trimester...
....
....

3. Past Medical History...
....
....

4. Present Surgical History. ....
....
....

5. Past Surgical History. ....
....
....

6. Family History. ....
....
....

7. Personal History. ....
....
....

OBSTETRICAL HISTORY

S.No.	Year	Abortion	Prem	F.T.	Type of Labour and Mode of Delivery	Gender	Live or Still Birth	Remark

ANTENATAL ATTENDANCES							
LMP.............................. EDD..Gestation at 1st visit.................. wk							
Date	Wt	BP	FHS	Weeks	Fundal Height	Presentation	Treatments and Remarks

GENERAL EXAMINATION

Poor/Fair/Good

Height: .... cms Weight:............................ Kgs

BP: mm Hg .... Temp: ....Pulse:..................... /Min Resp:........................./Min

Urine: Alb .... Sugar...

PHYSICAL EXAMINATION

HEAD: Hygiene...

Injury...

Surgery...

Infection ....

Any other ....

FACE: Expression...

Symmetry...

Chloasma ....

Scar...

EYES: Field of Vision...

Vision ....

Conjunctiva ....

Sclera. ....

Periorbital Oedema ....

Complaints if any ....

EARS: Hygiene..........

Hearing..........

Pain..........

Wax..........

Discharge..........

Surgery..........

Complaints if any..........

NOSE: Septal Deviation..........

Discharge..........

Bleeding..........

Polyp..........

Hygiene..........

Complaints if any..........

MOUTH: Lips: Colour.......... Texture..........

Stomatitis:..........

Hygiene:..........

Halitosis:..........

Tongue:..........

Teeth: Stain..........Symmetry..........Caries..........Extractions..........

Pain ....Fillings. ....

GUMS: Colour..........

Bleeding..........

Gingivitis..........

Complaints if any..........

NECK: Hygiene..........

Nodes..........

Glands..........

Thyroid..........

Jugular Veins..........

Scar..........

Complaints if any..........

CHEST: Shape..

Scar. ....

LIMBS: Upper-Symmetry..

Tremors..

Nails..

Hygiene..

Infection ....

Ulnar Nerve ....

Sub.Trochlear Node..

Axilla ....

Oedema..

Lower-Symmetry..

Hygiene..

Infection ....

Nails..

Oedema..

Varicose Veins..

BACK: Hygiene..

Deformity..

Pain..

Oedema..

OBSTETRICAL EXAMINATION

BREAST: Development..

Consistency ....

Symmetry..

Veins..

Areola ....

Primary..

Secondary ....

Montgomery's Tuberculosis ....

Nipples condition..

Colostrum ....

Lumps..

Axillary Nodes..

PERINEUM: Hygiene..

Discharge ....

Bleeding..

Pruritis ....

Infection..

Oedema ....

Complaints if any..

ABDOMEN

Measurements:

Fundal Height.. cms

Abdominal Girth.. cm

Gestational Age (by date)..

Inspection:

Shape..

Size ....

Hygiene..

Scars ....

Veins..

Fetal Movements..

Linea Nigra..

Striae ....

Palpation:

Fundal Palpation...

Rt. Lateral...

Lt. Lateral...

Pelvic Palpation...

Pawlick Grip...

Ausculation:

FHS...

Conclusion:

Lie...

Attitude...

Presentation...

Position...

Prest. Part: Eng/Not Engaged...

INVESTIGATION

INVESTIGATION BIOCHEMICAL										BIOPHYSICAL							
		Blood					Urine			USG							
S. No.	Date	Hb	Blood Group	HIV	VDRL	Blood Sugar	R	C	Stool	NST	BPP	FL/CRL	Placenta	Gest.Wks	LIQ	Anamoly

Any Other: ....

Treatment: Drugs...

Supportive: ....

DAILY OBSERVATION

Date	Temp	Pulse	Resp	BP	Weight	FSH	Urine output	Urine		Fundal HT	Abd. Girth	Kicks Count 4 hrly
								Albu	Sugar			

NURSING PROBLEM AND RELATED OBJECTIVE OF CARE

Actual Problem Nursing Problem..

....

....

....

....

....

Potential Problem Nursing Problem..

....

....

....

....

....

NURSING CARE PLAN

ASSESSMENT	NSG DIAGNOSIS	GOAL	PLANNING	IMPLEMENTATION

HEALTH EDUCATION

Date ....Topic...

Content

....

....

....

....

....

Teacher Signature..

ANTENATAL CARE STUDY

IDENTIFICATION DATA

Name of Mother...

Reg. No:...

Age: ....

Gravida: ....

Para:...

Diagnosis: ....

Date of Admission:..

Date of Discharge: ....

PAST MENSTRUAL HISTORY

LMP ....EDD ....Cycle...

HEALTH HISTORY

1. Past Obstetrical History...

....

....

2. Present Pregnancy History

- I-trimester ....

....

....

- II-trimester ....

....

....

- III-trimester..

....

....

3. Past Medical History..

....

....

4. Present Surgical History. ....

....

....

5. Past Surgical History. ....

....

....

6. Family History. ....

....

....

7. Personal History. ....

....

....

OBSTETRICAL HISTORY

S.No.	Year	Abortion	Prem	F.T.	Type of Labour and Mode of Delivery	Gender	Live or Still Birth	Remark

ANTENATAL ATTENDANCES

LMP............................ EDD...Gestation at 1st visit.................. wk

Date	Wt	BP	FHS	Weeks	Fundal Height	Presentation	Treatments and Remarks

GENERAL EXAMINATION

Poor/Fair/Good

Height: .... cms   Weight:............................ Kgs

BP: mm Hg ....   Temp: ....Pulse:...................... /Min   Resp:......................./Min

Urine: Alb .... Sugar...

PHYSICAL EXAMINATION

HEAD: Hygiene..

Injury..

Surgery..

Infection ....

Any other ....

FACE: Expression..

Symmetry..

Chloasma ....

Scar..

EYES: Field of Vision..

Vision ....

Conjunctiva ....

Sclera. ....

Periorbital Oedema ....

Complaints if any ....

EARS: Hygiene..........

Hearing..........

Pain..........

Wax..........

Discharge..........

Surgery..........

Complaints if any..........

NOSE: Septal Deviation..........

Discharge..........

Bleeding..........

Polyp..........

Hygiene..........

Complaints if any..........

MOUTH: Lips: Colour.......... Texture..........

Stomatitis:..........

Hygiene:..........

Halitosis:..........

Tongue:..........

Teeth: Stain..........Symmetry..........Caries..........Extractions..........

Pain ....Fillings. ....

GUMS: Colour..........

Bleeding..........

Gingivitis..........

Complaints if any..........

NECK: Hygiene..........

Nodes..........

Glands..........

Thyroid..........

Jugular Veins..........

Scar..........

Complaints if any..........

CHEST: Shape...

Scar. ....

LIMBS: Upper-Symmetry...

Tremors...

Nails...

Hygiene...

Infection ....

Ulnar Nerve ....

Sub.Trochlear Node...

Axilla ....

Oedema...

Lower-Symmetry...

Hygiene...

Infection ....

Nails...

Oedema...

Varicose Veins...

BACK: Hygiene...

Deformity...

Pain...

Oedema...

OBSTETRICAL EXAMINATION

BREAST: Development...

Consistency ....

Symmetry...

Veins...

Areola ....

Primary...

Secondary ....

Montgomery's Tuberculosis ....

Nipples condition..

Colostrum ....

Lumps..

Axillary Nodes..

PERINEUM: Hygiene..

Discharge ....

Bleeding..

Pruritis ....

Infection..

Oedema ....

Complaints if any...

ABDOMEN

Measurements:

Fundal Height.. cms

Abdominal Girth... cm

Gestational Age (by date)...

Inspection:

Shape..

Size ....

Hygiene..

Scars ....

Veins...

Fetal Movements...

Linea Nigra...

Striae ....

Palpation:

Fundal Palpation..........

Rt. Lateral..........

Lt. Lateral..........

Pelvic Palpation..........

Pawlick Grip..........

Ausculation:

FHS..........

Conclusion:

Lie..........

Attitude..........

Presentation..........

Position..........

Prest. Part: Eng/Not Engaged..........

INVESTIGATION

INVESTIGATION BIOCHEMICAL											BIOPHYSICAL							
		Blood					Urine			USG								
S. No.	Date	Hb	Blood Group	HIV	VDRL	Blood Sugar	R	C	Stool	NST	BPP	FL/CRL	Placenta	Gest.Wks	LIQ	Anamoly

Any Other: ....

Treatment: Drugs..........

Supportive: ....

DAILY OBSERVATION

Date	Temp	Pulse	Resp	BP	Weight	FSH	Urine output	Urine		Fundal HT	Abd. Girth	Kicks Count 4 hrly
								Albu	Sugar			

NURSING PROBLEM AND RELATED OBJECTIVE OF CARE

Actual Problem Nursing Problem..

....

....

....

....

....

Potential Problem Nursing Problem...

....

....

....

....

....

NURSING CARE PLAN

ASSESSMENT	NSG DIAGNOSIS	GOAL	PLANNING	IMPLEMENTATION

HEALTH EDUCATION

Date ....Topic..

Content

....

....

....

....

....

Teacher Signature..

ANTENATAL CARE STUDY

IDENTIFICATION DATA

Name of Mother..

Reg. No:..

Age: ....

Gravida: ....

Para:..

Diagnosis: ....

Date of Admission:..

Date of Discharge: ....

PAST MENSTRUAL HISTORY

LMP ....EDD ....Cycle...

HEALTH HISTORY

1. Past Obstetrical History..

....

....

2. Present Pregnancy History

- I-trimester..

....

....

- II-trimester..

....

....

- III-trimester...
....
....

3. Past Medical History...
....
....

4. Present Surgical History. ....
....
....

5. Past Surgical History. ....
....
....

6. Family History. ....
....
....

7. Personal History. ....
....
....

OBSTETRICAL HISTORY

S.No.	Year	Abortion	Prem	F.T.	Type of Labour and Mode of Delivery	Gender	Live or Still Birth	Remark

ANTENATAL ATTENDANCES

LMP............................ EDD...Gestation at 1st visit.................. wk

Date	Wt	BP	FHS	Weeks	Fundal Height	Presentation	Treatments and Remarks

GENERAL EXAMINATION

Poor/Fair/Good

Height: .... cms Weight:............................Kgs

BP: mm Hg .... Temp: ....Pulse:..................... /Min Resp:......................./Min

Urine: Alb .... Sugar...

PHYSICAL EXAMINATION

HEAD: Hygiene..

Injury..

Surgery..

Infection ....

Any other ....

FACE: Expression..

Symmetry..

Chloasma ....

Scar..

EYES: Field of Vision..

Vision ....

Conjunctiva ....

Sclera. ....

Periorbital Oedema ....

Complaints if any ....

EARS: Hygiene..

Hearing..

Pain..

Wax..

Discharge..

Surgery..

Complaints if any..

NOSE: Septal Deviation..

Discharge..

Bleeding..

Polyp..

Hygiene..

Complaints if any..

MOUTH: Lips: Colour.................................... Texture....................................

Stomatitis:..

Hygiene:..

Halitosis:..

Tongue:..

Teeth: Stain..............................Symmetry....................Caries..............................Extractions......................

Pain ....Fillings. ....

GUMS: Colour..

Bleeding..

Gingivitis..

Complaints if any..

NECK: Hygiene..

Nodes..

Glands..

Thyroid..

Jugular Veins..

Scar..

Complaints if any..

CHEST: Shape..........

Scar..........

LIMBS: Upper-Symmetry..........

Tremors..........

Nails..........

Hygiene..........

Infection..........

Ulnar Nerve..........

Sub.Trochlear Node..........

Axilla..........

Oedema..........

Lower-Symmetry..........

Hygiene..........

Infection..........

Nails..........

Oedema..........

Varicose Veins..........

BACK: Hygiene..........

Deformity..........

Pain..........

Oedema..........

OBSTETRICAL EXAMINATION

BREAST: Development..........

Consistency..........

Symmetry..........

Veins..........

Areola..........

Primary..........

Secondary ....

Montgomery's Tuberculosis ....

Nipples condition ....

Colostrum ....

Lumps ....

Axillary Nodes ....

PERINEUM: Hygiene ....

Discharge ....

Bleeding ....

Pruritis ....

Infection ....

Oedema ....

Complaints if any ....

ABDOMEN

Measurements:

Fundal Height .... cms

Abdominal Girth .... cm

Gestational Age (by date) ....

Inspection:

Shape ....

Size ....

Hygiene ....

Scars ....

Veins ....

Fetal Movements ....

Linea Nigra ....

Striae ....

Palpation:

Fundal Palpation..

Rt. Lateral..

Lt. Lateral..

Pelvic Palpation..

Pawlick Grip..

Ausculation:

FHS..

Conclusion:

Lie..

Attitude..

Presentation..

Position..

Prest. Part: Eng/Not Engaged..

INVESTIGATION

INVESTIGATION BIOCHEMICAL										BIOPHYSICAL						
S. No.	Date	Blood					Urine		Stool	USG						
		Hb	Blood Group	HIV	VDRL	Blood Sugar	R	C		NST	BPP	FL/CRL	Placenta	Gest.Wks	LIQ	Anamoly

Any Other: ....

Treatment: Drugs..

Supportive: ....

DAILY OBSERVATION

Date	Temp	Pulse	Resp	BP	Weight	FSH	Urine output	Urine		Fundal HT	Abd. Girth	Kicks Count 4 hrly
								Albu	Sugar			

NURSING PROBLEM AND RELATED OBJECTIVE OF CARE

Actual Problem Nursing Problem..

....

....

....

....

....

Potential Problem Nursing Problem..

....

....

....

....

....

NURSING CARE PLAN

ASSESSMENT	NSG DIAGNOSIS	GOAL	PLANNING	IMPLEMENTATION

HEALTH EDUCATION

Date ....Topic...

Content

....

....

....

....

....

Teacher Signature..

ANTENATAL CARE STUDY

IDENTIFICATION DATA

Name of Mother..

Reg. No:..

Age: ....

Gravida: ....

Para:..

Diagnosis: ....

Date of Admission:..

Date of Discharge: ....

PAST MENSTRUAL HISTORY

LMP ....EDD ....Cycle...

HEALTH HISTORY

1. Past Obstetrical History..

   ....

   ....

2. Present Pregnancy History

   - I-trimester..

     ....

     ....

   - II-trimester..

     ....

     ....

- III-trimester..

....

....

3. Past Medical History ....

....

....

4. Present Surgical History. ....

....

....

5. Past Surgical History. ....

....

....

6. Family History. ....

....

....

7. Personal History. ....

....

....

OBSTETRICAL HISTORY

S.No.	Year	Abortion	Prem	F.T.	Type of Labour and Mode of Delivery	Gender	Live or Still Birth	Remark

ANTENATAL ATTENDANCES

LMP............................ EDD..Gestation at 1st visit.................. wk

Date	Wt	BP	FHS	Weeks	Fundal Height	Presentation	Treatments and Remarks

GENERAL EXAMINATION

Poor/Fair/Good

Height: .... cms Weight:............................Kgs

BP: mm Hg .... Temp: ....Pulse:..................... /Min Resp:......................./Min

Urine: Alb .... Sugar...

PHYSICAL EXAMINATION

HEAD: Hygiene...

Injury...

Surgery...

Infection ....

Any other ....

FACE: Expression...

Symmetry...

Chloasma ....

Scar...

EYES: Field of Vision...

Vision ....

Conjunctiva ....

Sclera. ....

Periorbital Oedema ....

Complaints if any ....

EARS: Hygiene..

Hearing..

Pain..

Wax..

Discharge..

Surgery..

Complaints if any..

NOSE: Septal Deviation..

Discharge..

Bleeding..

Polyp..

Hygiene..

Complaints if any..

MOUTH: Lips: Colour.................................... Texture....................................

Stomatitis:..

Hygiene:..

Halitosis:..

Tongue:..

Teeth: Stain..............................Symmetry..................Caries..............................Extractions......................

Pain ....Fillings. ....

GUMS: Colour..

Bleeding..

Gingivitis..

Complaints if any..

NECK: Hygiene..

Nodes..

Glands..

Thyroid..

Jugular Veins..

Scar..

Complaints if any..

CHEST: Shape..

Scar. ....

LIMBS: Upper-Symmetry..

Tremors..

Nails..

Hygiene..

Infection ....

Ulnar Nerve ....

Sub.Trochlear Node..

Axilla ....

Oedema..

Lower-Symmetry..

Hygiene..

Infection ....

Nails..

Oedema..

Varicose Veins..

BACK: Hygiene..

Deformity..

Pain..

Oedema..

OBSTETRICAL EXAMINATION

BREAST: Development..

Consistency ....

Symmetry..

Veins..

Areola ....

Primary..

Secondary ....

Montgomery's Tuberculosis ....

Nipples condition ....

Colostrum ....

Lumps ....

Axillary Nodes ....

PERINEUM: Hygiene ....

Discharge ....

Bleeding ....

Pruritis ....

Infection ....

Oedema ....

Complaints if any ....

ABDOMEN

Measurements:

Fundal Height .... cms

Abdominal Girth .... cm

Gestational Age (by date) ....

Inspection:

Shape ....

Size ....

Hygiene ....

Scars ....

Veins ....

Fetal Movements ....

Linea Nigra ....

Striae ....

Palpation:

Fundal Palpation..........

Rt. Lateral..........

Lt. Lateral..........

Pelvic Palpation..........

Pawlick Grip..........

Ausculation:

FHS..........

Conclusion:

Lie..........

Attitude..........

Presentation..........

Position..........

Prest. Part: Eng/Not Engaged..........

INVESTIGATION

INVESTIGATION BIOCHEMICAL										BIOPHYSICAL							
		Blood					Urine			USG							
S. No.	Date	Hb	Blood Group	HIV	VDRL	Blood Sugar	R	C	Stool	NST	BPP	FL/CRL	Placenta	Gest.Wks	LIQ	Anamoly

Any Other: ....

Treatment: Drugs..........

Supportive: ....

DAILY OBSERVATION

Date	Temp	Pulse	Resp	BP	Weight	FSH	Urine output	Urine		Fundal HT	Abd. Girth	Kicks Count 4 hrly
								Albu	Sugar			

NURSING PROBLEM AND RELATED OBJECTIVE OF CARE

Actual Problem Nursing Problem...

....

....

....

....

....

Potential Problem Nursing Problem...

....

....

....

....

....

NURSING CARE PLAN

ASSESSMENT	NSG DIAGNOSIS	GOAL	PLANNING	IMPLEMENTATION

HEALTH EDUCATION

Date ....Topic...

Content

....

....

....

....

....

Teacher Signature..

ANTENATAL CARE STUDY

IDENTIFICATION DATA

Name of Mother..

Reg. No:..

Age: ....

Gravida: ....

Para:...

Diagnosis: ....

Date of Admission:..

Date of Discharge: ....

PAST MENSTRURAL HISTORY

LMP ....EDD ....Cycle..

HEALTH HISTORY

1. Past Obstetrical History...

   ....

   ....

2. Present Pregnancy History

   - I-trimester ....

     ....

     ....

   - II-trimester...

     ....

     ....

- III-trimester..
....
....

3. Past Medical History..
....
....

4. Present Surgical History. ....
....
....

5. Past Surgical History. ....
....
....

6. Family History. ....
....
....

7. Personal History. ....
....
....

OBSTETRICAL HISTORY

S.No.	Year	Abortion	Prem	F.T.	Type of Labour and Mode of Delivery	Gender	Live or Still Birth	Remark

ANTENATAL ATTENDANCES

LMP.............................. EDD..Gestation at 1st visit.................. wk

Date	Wt	BP	FHS	Weeks	Fundal Height	Presentation	Treatments and Remarks

GENERAL EXAMINATION

Poor/Fair/Good

Height: .... cms Weight:............................. Kgs

BP: mm Hg .... Temp: ....Pulse:..................... /Min Resp:........................./Min

Urine: Alb .... Sugar..

PHYSICAL EXAMINATION

HEAD: Hygiene..

Injury..

Surgery..

Infection ....

Any other ....

FACE: Expression..

Symmetry..

Chloasma ....

Scar..

EYES: Field of Vision..

Vision ....

Conjunctiva ....

Sclera. ....

Periorbital Oedema ....

Complaints if any ....

EARS: Hygiene..

Hearing..

Pain..

Wax..

Discharge..

Surgery..

Complaints if any..

NOSE: Septal Deviation..

Discharge..

Bleeding..

Polyp..

Hygiene..

Complaints if any..

MOUTH: Lips: Colour........................ Texture........................

Stomatitis:..

Hygiene:..

Halitosis:..

Tongue:..

Teeth: Stain....................Symmetry....................Caries....................Extractions....................

Pain ....Fillings. ....

GUMS: Colour..

Bleeding..

Gingivitis..

Complaints if any..

NECK: Hygiene..

Nodes..

Glands..

Thyroid..

Jugular Veins..

Scar..

Complaints if any..

CHEST: Shape..

Scar. ....

LIMBS: Upper-Symmetry..

Tremors..

Nails..

Hygiene..

Infection ....

Ulnar Nerve ....

Sub.Trochlear Node..

Axilla ....

Oedema..

Lower-Symmetry..

Hygiene..

Infection ....

Nails..

Oedema..

Varicose Veins..

BACK: Hygiene..

Deformity..

Pain..

Oedema..

OBSTETRICAL EXAMINATION

BREAST: Development..

Consistency ....

Symmetry..

Veins..

Areola ....

Primary..

Secondary ....

Montgomery's Tuberculosis ....

Nipples condition ....

Colostrum ....

Lumps ....

Axillary Nodes ....

PERINEUM: Hygiene ....

Discharge ....

Bleeding ....

Pruritis ....

Infection ....

Oedema ....

Complaints if any ....

ABDOMEN

Measurements:

Fundal Height .... cms

Abdominal Girth .... cm

Gestational Age (by date) ....

Inspection:

Shape ....

Size ....

Hygiene ....

Scars ....

Veins ....

Fetal Movements ....

Linea Nigra ....

Striae ....

Palpation:

Fundal Palpation..

Rt. Lateral..

Lt. Lateral..

Pelvic Palpation..

Pawlick Grip..

Ausculation:

FHS..

Conclusion:

Lie..

Attitude..

Presentation..

Position..

Prest. Part: Eng/Not Engaged..

INVESTIGATION

INVESTIGATION BIOCHEMICAL											BIOPHYSICAL							
S. No.	Date	Blood					Urine		Stool	USG								
		Hb	Blood Group	HIV	VDRL	Blood Sugar	R	C		NST	BPP	FL/CRL	Placenta	Gest.Wks	LIQ	Anamoly

Any Other: ....

Treatment: Drugs..

Supportive: ....

DAILY OBSERVATION

Date	Temp	Pulse	Resp	BP	Weight	FSH	Urine output	Urine		Fundal HT	Abd. Girth	Kicks Count 4 hrly
								Albu	Sugar			

NURSING PROBLEM AND RELATED OBJECTIVE OF CARE

Actual Problem Nursing Problem..

....

....

....

....

....

Potential Problem Nursing Problem..

....

....

....

....

....

NURSING CARE PLAN

ASSESSMENT	NSG DIAGNOSIS	GOAL	PLANNING	IMPLEMENTATION

HEALTH EDUCATION

Date .... Topic...

Content

....

....

....

....

....

Teacher Signature..

ANTENATAL CARE STUDY

IDENTIFICATION DATA

Name of Mother..

Reg. No:..

Age: ....

Gravida: ....

Para:...

Diagnosis: ....

Date of Admission:...

Date of Discharge: ....

PAST MENSTRUAL HISTORY

LMP ....EDD ....Cycle..

HEALTH HISTORY

1. Past Obstetrical History...

   ....

   ....

2. Present Pregnancy History

   - I-trimester ....

     ....

     ....

   - II-trimester...

     ....

     ....

- III-trimester..
....
....

3. Past Medical History..
....
....

4. Present Surgical History. ....
....
....

5. Past Surgical History. ....
....
....

6. Family History. ....
....
....

7. Personal History. ....
....
....

OBSTETRICAL HISTORY

S.No.	Year	Abortion	Prem	F.T.	Type of Labour and Mode of Delivery	Gender	Live or Still Birth	Remark

ANTENATAL ATTENDANCES

LMP............................ EDD...Gestation at 1st visit.................. wk

Date	Wt	BP	FHS	Weeks	Fundal Height	Presentation	Treatments and Remarks

GENERAL EXAMINATION

Poor/Fair/Good

Height: .... cms Weight:............................ Kgs

BP: mm Hg .... Temp: ....Pulse:..................... /Min Resp:........................../Min

Urine: Alb .... Sugar...

PHYSICAL EXAMINATION

HEAD: Hygiene...

Injury...

Surgery...

Infection ....

Any other ....

FACE: Expression...

Symmetry...

Chloasma ....

Scar...

EYES: Field of Vision...

Vision ....

Conjunctiva ....

Sclera. ....

Periorbital Oedema ....

Complaints if any ....

EARS: Hygiene..

Hearing..

Pain..

Wax..

Discharge..

Surgery..

Complaints if any..

NOSE: Septal Deviation..

Discharge..

Bleeding..

Polyp..

Hygiene..

Complaints if any..

MOUTH: Lips: Colour.................... Texture....................

Stomatitis:..

Hygiene:..

Halitosis:..

Tongue:..

Teeth: Stain....................Symmetry....................Caries....................Extractions....................

Pain ....Fillings. ....

GUMS: Colour..

Bleeding..

Gingivitis..

Complaints if any..

NECK: Hygiene..

Nodes..

Glands..

Thyroid..

Jugular Veins..

Scar..

Complaints if any..

CHEST: Shape...

Scar. ....

LIMBS: Upper-Symmetry...

Tremors...

Nails...

Hygiene...

Infection ....

Ulnar Nerve ....

Sub.Trochlear Node...

Axilla ....

Oedema...

Lower-Symmetry...

Hygiene...

Infection ....

Nails...

Oedema...

Varicose Veins...

BACK: Hygiene...

Deformity...

Pain...

Oedema...

OBSTETRICAL EXAMINATION

BREAST: Development...

Consistency ....

Symmetry...

Veins...

Areola ....

Primary...

Secondary ....

Montgomery's Tuberculosis ....

Nipples condition..

Colostrum ....

Lumps..

Axillary Nodes..

PERINEUM: Hygiene..

Discharge ....

Bleeding..

Pruritis ....

Infection..

Oedema ....

Complaints if any..

ABDOMEN

Measurements:

Fundal Height..cms

Abdominal Girth.. cm

Gestational Age (by date)..

Inspection:

Shape..

Size ....

Hygiene..

Scars ....

Veins..

Fetal Movements..

Linea Nigra..

Striae ....

Palpation:

Fundal Palpation..

Rt. Lateral..

Lt. Lateral..

Pelvic Palpation..

Pawlick Grip..

Ausculation:

FHS..

Conclusion:

Lie..

Attitude..

Presentation..

Position..

Prest. Part: Eng/Not Engaged..

INVESTIGATION

INVESTIGATION BIOCHEMICAL											BIOPHYSICAL						
		Blood					Urine			USG							
S. No.	Date	Hb	Blood Group	HIV	VDRL	Blood Sugar	R	C	Stool	NST	BPP	FL/CRL	Placenta	Gest.Wks	LIQ	Anamoly	

Any Other: ....

Treatment: Drugs..

Supportive: ....

DAILY OBSERVATION

Date	Temp	Pulse	Resp	BP	Weight	FSH	Urine output	Urine		Fundal HT	Abd. Girth	Kicks Count 4 hrly
								Albu	Sugar			

NURSING PROBLEM AND RELATED OBJECTIVE OF CARE

Actual Problem Nursing Problem..

....

....

....

....

....

Potential Problem Nursing Problem..

....

....

....

....

....

NURSING CARE PLAN

ASSESSMENT	NSG DIAGNOSIS	GOAL	PLANNING	IMPLEMENTATION

HEALTH EDUCATION

Date ....Topic...

Content

....

....

....

....

....

Teacher Signature..

CONDUCTED CARE STUDY

IDENTIFICATION DATA

Name of the Mother:..

Reg.No:..

Age:..

Gravida:..

Parity:..

Date of Admission and Time:..

Date of Delivery and Time:..

Date of Discharge:..

PAST MENSTRUAL HISTORY

LMP ....EDD ....Cycle..

HEALTH HISTORY

1. Past Obstetrical History..

   ....

   ....

2. Present Pregnancy History

   - I-trimester ....

     ....

     ....

   - II-trimester..

     ....

     ....

   - III-trimester..

     ....

     ....

3. Past Medical History ....

....

....

4. Present Surgical History. ....

....

....

5. Past Surgical History. ....

....

....

6. Family History. ....

....

....

7. Personal History. ....

....

....

OBSTETRICAL HISTORY

S.No.	Year	Abortion	Prem	F.T.	Type of Labour and Mode of Delivery	Gender	Live or Still Birth	Remark

INVESTIGATION

USG Date: ....Finding: BPD..

FL/CRL..

Blood Group: .... Hb: .... Urine: ALB....................... Placenta..

RH Factor: .... VDRL:..................................... Sug.................... ....Gest. Wks..

Liquor..

Anamoly..

ANTENATAL ATTENDANCES

LMP............................ EDD..Gestation at 1st visit.................. wk

Date	Wt	BP	FHS	Weeks	Fundal height	Presentation	Treatments and Remarks

Labour Ward Admission Notes:

Admitted on:..at .... AM/PM

Contraction Commenced on: ....at .... AM/PM

Period of Gestation:..weeks

Height of Fundus..cms.

Presentation:..

Position: ....

Engaged /Not Engaged:

FHS:.. /min

Bladder: Voided/Catheter

Bowel: SE Given/Not Given (Reason)

Remarks if Any:...

LABOUR RECORD : 1st STAGE

I.	**OBSERVATION**										
	UTERINE CONTRATION										
	a. Frequency in 10 mins										
	b. Duration in Secs										
	c. Intensity										
II.	**PER VAGINAL EXAM**										
	a. Cervical Dilatation										
	b. Cer. Effacement										
	c. Membranes										
	d. Presentation Part										
	e. Station										
	f. Position of Occiput										
	PARAMETERS										
	a. FHS/min										
III.	b. Pulse/min										
	c. BP										
	d. Urine output										
IV.	**MEDICATION**										
V.	**SUPPORTIVE TREATMENT**										

IInd Stage

Membranes Ruptured at..AM/PM Spont/Artificial

Colour of Liqour..

Full Dilation /Explusive Cont Began at ....AM/PM On..

MOTHER:

Perineum: Rigid/Lax

Episiotomy: Given /Not Given

NEONATE:

Born at: ....AM/PM

On:..

Gender: Male/Female

Apgar Score 1min:..

5 min: ....

Complication:

Treatment: Airway:.......................................

Eyes:..

Cord: ....

IIIrd Stage

a. Placenta and Membranes:

Delivered at.. AM/PM

Complete/Incomplete

Cord Insertion: Central/Marginal/Velamentous

Cord Length: ....(Inches)

Weight:...

b. Condition of Uterus:

c. PERINEUM: Episiotomy/Tear Laceration

Repair:..No.of Sutures ....No.of Catgut

d. Drugs given: ....

e. Approximate blood loss ....ml

PARTOGRAPH

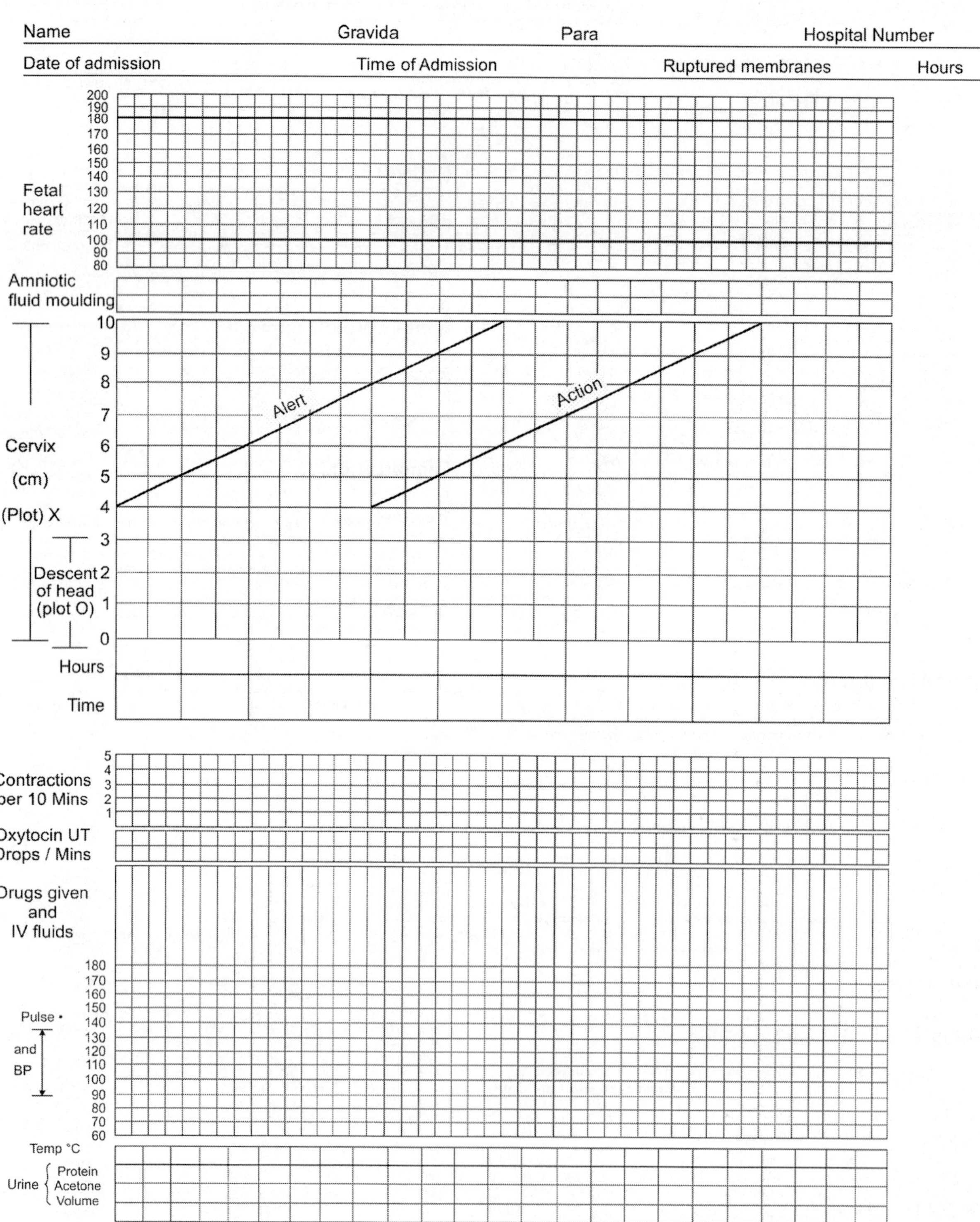
Name
Gravida
Para
Hospital Number
Date of admission
Time of Admission
Ruptured membranes
Hours
Fetal heart rate
200 190 180 170 160 150 140 130 120 110 100 90 80
Amniotic fluid moulding
Cervix (cm) (Plot) X
10 9 8 7 6 5 4 3 2 1 0
Alert
Action
Descent of head (plot O)
Hours
Time
Contractions per 10 Mins
5 4 3 2 1
Oxytocin UT Drops / Mins
Drugs given and IV fluids
Pulse •
and BP
180 170 160 150 140 130 120 110 100 90 80 70 60
Temp °C
Urine
Protein
Acetone
Volume

LABOUR SUMMARY

Type of labour: Spont/Induced

Mode of delivery: Vaginal/Instrument

Length of Labour:

1st stage .... Hrs .... Mins

2nd stage .... Hrs .... Mins

3rd stage .... Hrs .... Mins

Delivered by: ....

CONDUCTED CARE STUDY

IDENTIFICATION DATA

Name of the Mother:..........

Reg.No:..........

Age:..........

Gravida:..........

Parity:..........

Date of Admission and Time:..........

Date of Delivery and Time:..........

Date of Discharge:..........

PAST MENSTRUAL HISTORY

LMP ....EDD ....Cycle..........

HEALTH HISTORY

1. Past Obstetrical History..........

   ....

   ....

2. Present Pregnancy History

   - I-trimester ....

     ....

     ....

   - II-trimester ....

     ....

     ....

   - III-trimester..........

     ....

     ....

3. Past Medical History ....

....

....

4. Present Surgical History. ....

....

....

5. Past Surgical History. ....

....

....

6. Family History. ....

....

....

7. Personal History. ....

....

....

OBSTETRICAL HISTORY

S.No.	Year	Abortion	Prem	F.T.	Type of Labour and Mode of Delivery	Gender	Live or Still Birth	Remark

INVESTIGATION

USG Date: ....Finding: BPD..

FL/CRL..

Blood Group: .... Hb: .... Urine: ALB .... Placenta..

RH Factor: .... VDRL:.................................... Sug.................. .... Gest. Wks...

Liquor..

Anamoly..

ANTENATAL ATTENDANCES

LMP.............................. EDD...Gestation at 1st visit................... wk

Date	Wt	BP	FHS	Weeks	Fundal height	Presentation	Treatments and Remarks

Labour Ward Admission Notes:

Admitted on:...at .... AM/PM

Contraction Commenced on: ....at .... AM/PM

Period of Gestation:..weeks

Height of Fundus..cms.

Presentation:...

Position: ....

Engaged /Not Engaged:

FHS:.. /min

Bladder: Voided/Catheter

Bowel: SE Given/Not Given (Reason)

Remarks if Any:..

LABOUR RECORD : 1st STAGE

I.	**OBSERVATION**										
	UTERINE CONTRATION										
	a. Frequency in 10 mins										
	b. Duration in Secs										
	c. Intensity										
II.	**PER VAGINAL EXAM**										
	a. Cervical Dilatation										
	b. Cer. Effacement										
	c. Membranes										
	d. Presentation Part										
	e. Station										
	f. Position of Occiput										
III.	**PARAMETERS**										
	e. FHS/min										
	f. Pulse/min										
	g. BP										
	h. Urine output										
IV.	**MEDICATION**										
V.	**SUPPORTIVE TREATMENT**										

IInd Stage

Membranes Ruptured at..AM/PM Spont/Artificial

Colour of Liqour..

Full Dilation /Explusive Cont Began at ....AM/PM On...

MOTHER:

Perineum: Rigid/Lax

Episiotomy: Given /Not Given

NEONATE:

Born at: ....AM/PM

On:..

Gender: Male/Female

Apgar Score 1min: ....

5 min: ....

Complication:

Treatment: Airway: ....

Eyes:..

Cord:...

IIIrd Stage

a. **Placenta and Membranes:**

Delivered at.. AM/PM

Complete/Incomplete

Cord Insertion: Central/Marginal/Velamentous

Cord Length: .... (Inches)

Weight:...

b. **Condition of Uterus:**

c. **PERINEUM:** Episiotomy/Tear Laceration

Repair:...No.of Sutures ....No.of Catgut

d. **Drugs given:** ....

e. Approximate blood loss ....ml

PARTOGRAPH

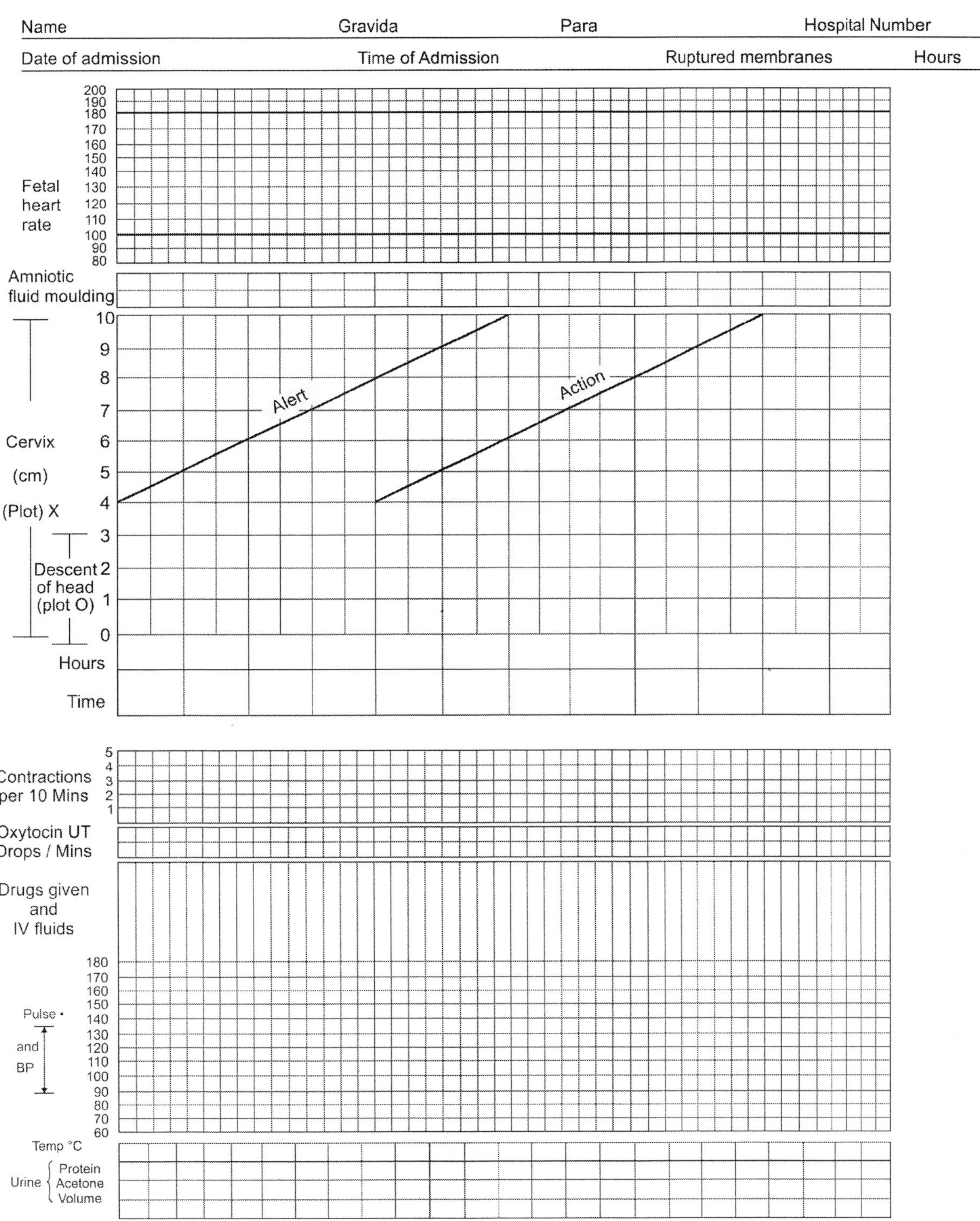

Name
Gravida
Para
Hospital Number
Date of admission
Time of Admission
Ruptured membranes
Hours
Fetal heart rate
200
190
180
170
160
150
140
130
120
110
100
90
80
Amniotic fluid moulding
Cervix (cm) (Plot) X
10
9
8
7
6
5
4
3
2
1
0
Alert
Action
Descent of head (plot O)
Hours
Time
Contractions per 10 Mins
5
4
3
2
1
Oxytocin UT Drops / Mins
Drugs given and IV fluids
Pulse •
and BP
180
170
160
150
140
130
120
110
100
90
80
70
60
Temp °C
Urine
Protein
Acetone
Volume

LABOUR SUMMARY

Type of labour: Spont/Induced

Mode of delivery: Vaginal/Instrument

Length of Labour:

1st stage .... Hrs .... Mins

2nd stage .... Hrs .... Mins

3rd stage .... Hrs .... Mins

Delivered by: ....

CONDUCTED CARE STUDY

IDENTIFICATION DATA

Name of the Mother:..

Reg.No: ....

Age:..

Gravida: ....

Parity:..

Date of Admission and Time: ....

Date of Delivery and Time:..

Date of Discharge:..

PAST MENSTRUAL HISTORY

LMP ....EDD ....Cycle...

HEALTH HISTORY

1. Past Obstetrical History..

....

....

2. Present Pregnancy History

- I-trimester ....

....

....

- II-trimester..

....

....

- III-trimester..

....

....

3. Past Medical History ....

....

....

4. Present Surgical History. ....

....

....

5. Past Surgical History. ....

....

....

6. Family History. ....

....

....

7. Personal History. ....

....

....

OBSTETRICAL HISTORY

S.No.	Year	Abortion	Prem	F.T.	Type of Labour and Mode of Delivery	Gender	Live or Still Birth	Remark

INVESTIGATION

USG Date: ....Finding: BPD..

FL/CRL..

Blood Group: .... Hb: .... Urine: ALB .... Placenta..

RH Factor: .... VDRL:.................................... Sug.................. .... Gest. Wks..

Liquor..

Anamoly..

ANTENATAL ATTENDANCES

LMP............................ EDD..Gestation at 1st visit.................. wk

Date	Wt	BP	FHS	Weeks	Fundal height	Presentation	Treatments and Remarks

Labour Ward Admission Notes:

Admitted on:..at .... AM/PM

Contraction Commenced on: ....at .... AM/PM

Period of Gestation:...weeks

Height of Fundus...cms.

Presentation:...

Position: ....

Engaged /Not Engaged:

FHS:... /min

Bladder: Voided/Catheter

Bowel: SE Given/Not Given (Reason)

Remarks if Any:...

LABOUR RECORD : 1st STAGE

I.	**OBSERVATION**										
	UTERINE CONTRATION										
	a. Frequency in 10 mins										
	b. Duration in Secs										
	c. Intensity										
II.	**PER VAGINAL EXAM**										
	a. Cervical Dilatation										
	b. Cer. Effacement										
	c. Membranes										
	d. Presentation Part										
	e. Station										
	f. Position of Occiput										
	PARAMETERS										
	i. FHS/min										
III.	j. Pulse/min										
	k. BP										
	l. Urine output										
IV.	**MEDICATION**										
V.	**SUPPORTIVE TREATMENT**										

IInd Stage

Membranes Ruptured at...AM/PM Spont/Artificial

Colour of Liqour...

Full Dilation /Explusive Cont Began at ....AM/PM On..

MOTHER:

Perineum: Rigid/Lax

Episiotomy: Given /Not Given

NEONATE:

Born at: ....AM/PM

On:..

Gender: Male/Female

Apgar Score 1min:..

5 min: ....

Complication:

Treatment: Airway:..

Eyes:...

Cord:...

IIIrd Stage

a. Placenta and Membranes:

Delivered at... AM/PM

Complete/Incomplete

Cord Insertion: Central/Marginal/Velamentous

Cord Length: .... (Inches)

Weight:..

b. Condition of Uterus:

c. PERINEUM: Episiotomy/Tear Laceration

Repair:...No.of Sutures ....No.of Catgut

d. Drugs given: ....

e. Approximate blood loss ....ml

PARTOGRAPH

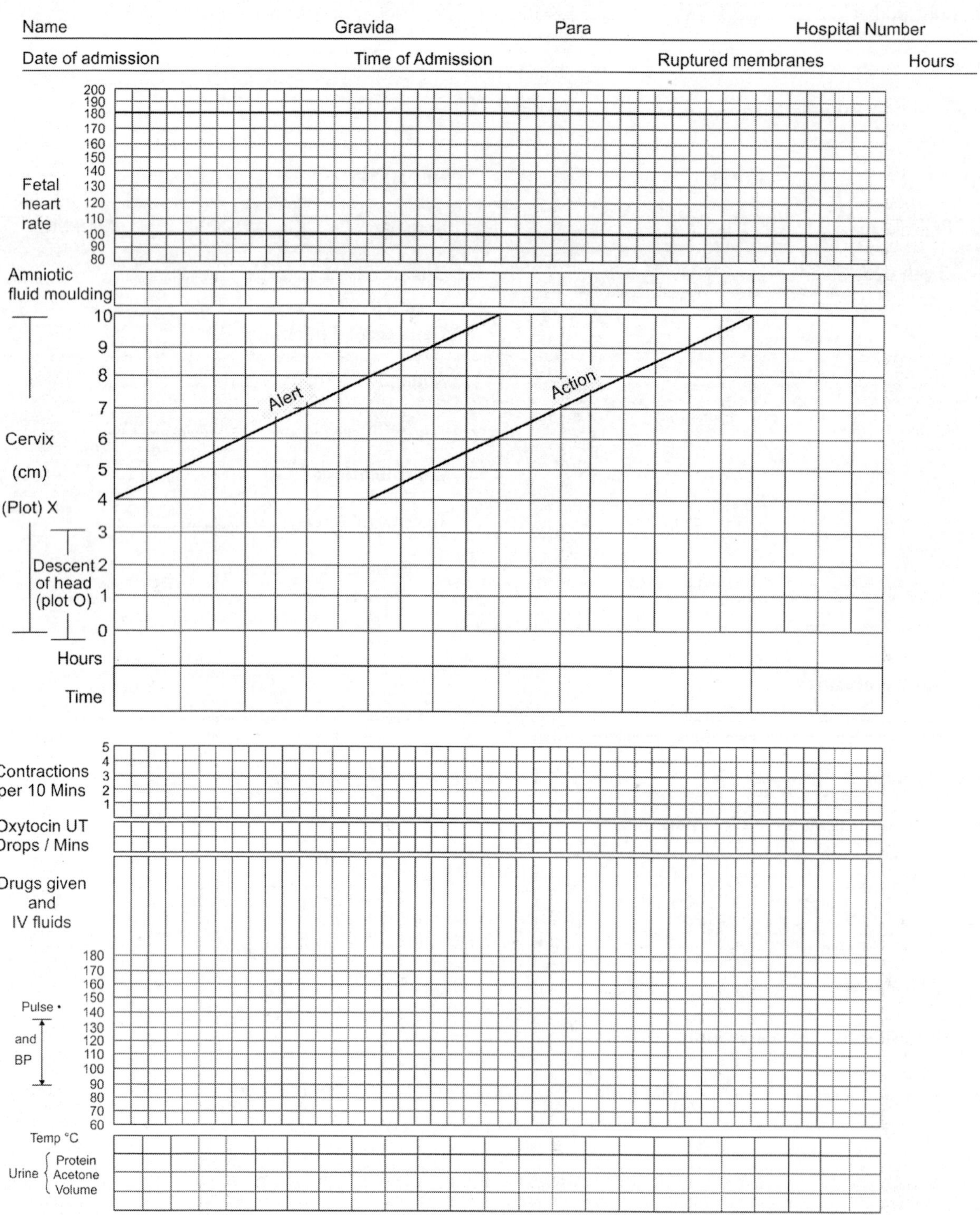
Name
Gravida
Para
Hospital Number
Date of admission
Time of Admission
Ruptured membranes
Hours
200
190
180
170
160
150
140
Fetal heart rate
130
120
110
100
90
80
Amniotic fluid moulding
10
9
8
7
Cervix (cm) (Plot) X
6
5
4
3
Descent of head (plot O)
2
1
0
Alert
Action
Hours
Time
Contractions per 10 Mins
5
4
3
2
1
Oxytocin UT Drops / Mins
Drugs given and IV fluids
Pulse •
and BP
180
170
160
150
140
130
120
110
100
90
80
70
60
Temp °C
Urine
Protein
Acetone
Volume

LABOUR SUMMARY

Type of labour: Spont/Induced

Mode of delivery: Vaginal/Instrument

Length of Labour:

1st stage .... Hrs .... Mins

2nd stage .... Hrs .... Mins

3rd stage .... Hrs .... Mins

Delivered by: ....

CONDUCTED CARE STUDY

IDENTIFICATION DATA

Name of the Mother:..

Reg.No:..

Age:..

Gravida:..

Parity:..

Date of Admission and Time:..

Date of Delivery and Time:..

Date of Discharge:..

PAST MENSTRUAL HISTORY

LMP ....EDD ....Cycle...

HEALTH HISTORY

1. Past Obstetrical History..

....

....

2. Present Pregnancy History

- I-trimester..

....

....

- II-trimester..

....

....

- III-trimester..

....

....

3. Past Medical History ....

....

....

4. Present Surgical History. ....

....

....

5. Past Surgical History. ....

....

....

6. Family History. ....

....

....

7. Personal History. ....

....

....

OBSTETRICAL HISTORY

S.No.	Year	Abortion	Prem	F.T.	Type of Labour and Mode of Delivery	Gender	Live or Still Birth	Remark

INVESTIGATION

USG Date: ....Finding: BPD...

FL/CRL..

Blood Group: .... Hb: .... Urine: ALB .... Placenta...

RH Factor: .... VDRL:.................................... Sug.................. ....Gest. Wks ....

Liquor ....

Anamoly ....

ANTENATAL ATTENDANCES							
LMP.............................. EDD...Gestation at 1st visit................... wk							
Date	Wt	BP	FHS	Weeks	Fundal height	Presentation	Treatments and Remarks

Labour Ward Admission Notes:

Admitted on:...at .... AM/PM

Contraction Commenced on: ....at .... AM/PM

Period of Gestation:..weeks

Height of Fundus...cms.

Presentation:...

Position: ....

Engaged /Not Engaged:

FHS:.. /min

Bladder: Voided/Catheter

Bowel: SE Given/Not Given (Reason)

Remarks if Any:...

LABOUR RECORD : 1st STAGE

I.	**OBSERVATION**										
	UTERINE CONTRATION										
	a. Frequency in 10 mins										
	b. Duration in Secs										
	c. Intensity										
II.	**PER VAGINAL EXAM**										
	a. Cervical Dilatation										
	b. Cer. Effacement										
	c. Membranes										
	d. Presentation Part										
	e. Station										
	f. Position of Occiput										
	PARAMETERS										
	m. FHS/min										
III.	n. Pulse/min										
	o. BP										
	p. Urine output										
IV.	**MEDICATION**										
V.	**SUPPORTIVE TREATMENT**										

IInd Stage

Membranes Ruptured at...AM/PM Spont/Artificial

Colour of Liqour..

Full Dilation /Explusive Cont Began at ....AM/PM On..

MOTHER:

Perineum: Rigid/Lax

Episiotomy: Given /Not Given

NEONATE:

Born at: ....AM/PM

On:..

Gender: Male/Female

Apgar Score 1min: ....

5 min: ....

Complication:

Treatment: Airway: ....

Eyes:..

Cord: ....

IIIrd Stage

a. Placenta and Membranes:

Delivered at... AM/PM

Complete/Incomplete

Cord Insertion: Central/Marginal/Velamentous

Cord Length: .... (Inches)

Weight:..

b. Condition of Uterus:

c. PERINEUM: Episiotomy/Tear Laceration

Repair:..No.of Sutures ....No.of Catgut

d. Drugs given: ....

e. Approximate blood loss ....ml

PARTOGRAPH

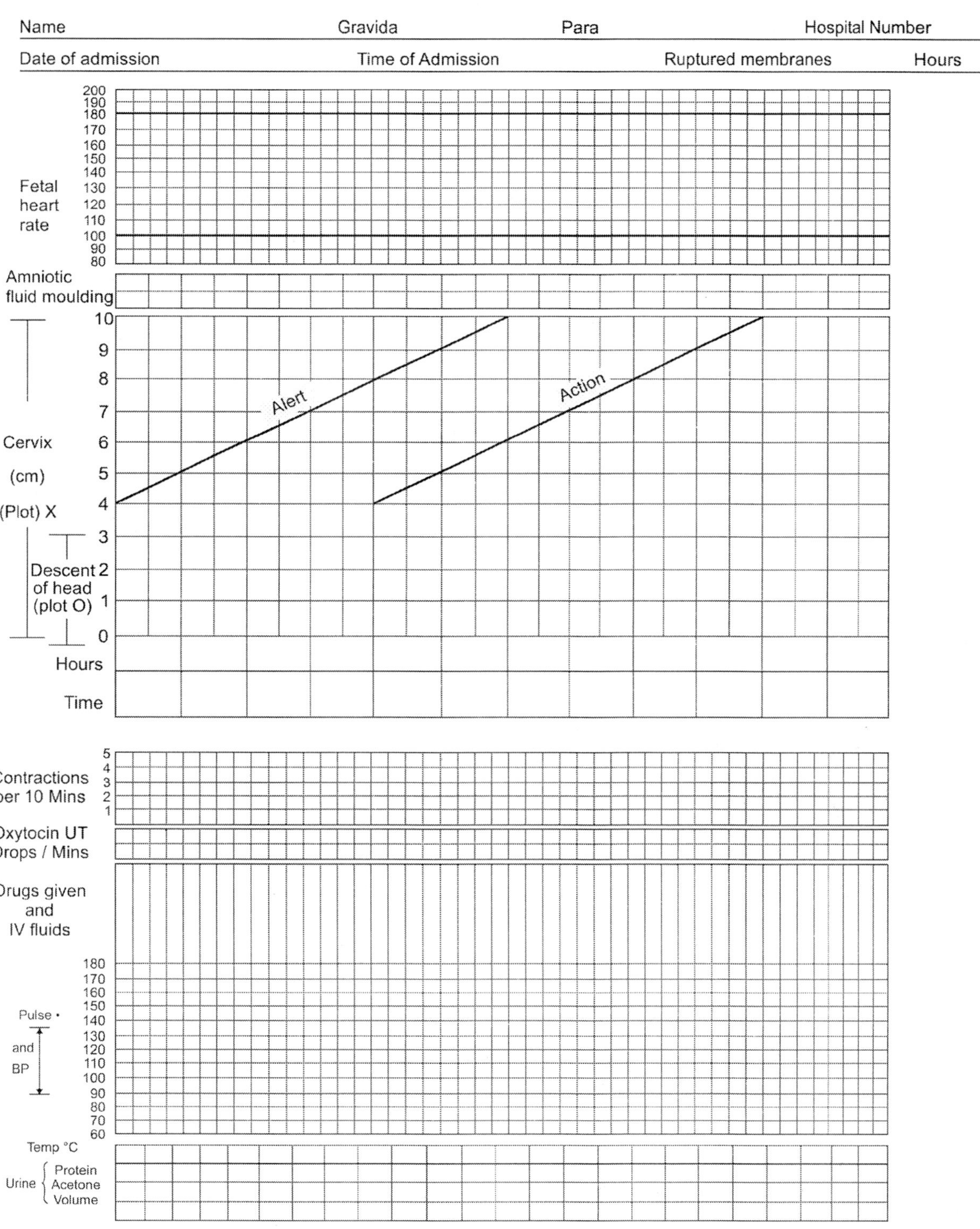
Name
Gravida
Para
Hospital Number
Date of admission
Time of Admission
Ruptured membranes
Hours
Fetal heart rate
200
190
180
170
160
150
140
130
120
110
100
90
80
Amniotic fluid moulding
Cervix (cm) (Plot) X
10
9
8
7
6
5
4
3
2
1
0
Alert
Action
Descent of head (plot O)
Hours
Time
Contractions per 10 Mins
5
4
3
2
1
Oxytocin UT Drops / Mins
Drugs given and IV fluids
Pulse •
and BP
180
170
160
150
140
130
120
110
100
90
80
70
60
Temp °C
Urine
Protein
Acetone
Volume

LABOUR SUMMARY

Type of labour: Spont/Induced

Mode of delivery: Vaginal/Instrument

Length of Labour:

1st stage .... Hrs .... Mins

2nd stage .... Hrs .... Mins

3rd stage .... Hrs .... Mins

Delivered by: ....

CONDUCTED CARE STUDY

IDENTIFICATION DATA

Name of the Mother:..

Reg.No: ....

Age:...

Gravida: ....

Parity: ....

Date of Admission and Time: ....

Date of Delivery and Time:...

Date of Discharge:...

PAST MENSTRUAL HISTORY

LMP ....EDD ....Cycle..

HEALTH HISTORY

1. Past Obstetrical History...

   ....

   ....

2. Present Pregnancy History
   - I-trimester ....

     ....

     ....
   - II-trimester...

     ....

     ....
   - III-trimester...

     ....

     ....

3. Past Medical History ....

....

....

4. Present Surgical History. ....

....

....

5. Past Surgical History. ....

....

....

6. Family History. ....

....

....

7. Personal History. ....

....

....

OBSTETRICAL HISTORY

S.No.	Year	Abortion	Prem	F.T.	Type of Labour and Mode of Delivery	Gender	Live or Still Birth	Remark

INVESTIGATION

USG Date: ....Finding: BPD...

FL/CRL..

Blood Group: .... Hb: .... Urine: ALB .... Placenta ....

RH Factor: .... VDRL:.................................... Sug.................... ....Gest. Wks ....

Liquor ....

Anamoly ....

ANTENATAL ATTENDANCES

LMP............................ EDD...Gestation at 1st visit.................. wk

Date	Wt	BP	FHS	Weeks	Fundal height	Presentation	Treatments and Remarks

Labour Ward Admission Notes:

Admitted on:...at ....AM/PM

Contraction Commenced on: ....at ....AM/PM

Period of Gestation:...weeks

Height of Fundus...cms.

Presentation:..

Position: ....

Engaged /Not Engaged:

FHS:.. /min

Bladder: Voided/Catheter

Bowel: SE Given/Not Given (Reason)

Remarks if Any:..

LABOUR RECORD : 1st STAGE

I.	**OBSERVATION**										
	UTERINE CONTRATION										
	a. Frequency in 10 mins										
	b. Duration in Secs										
	c. Intensity										
II.	**PER VAGINAL EXAM**										
	a. Cervical Dilatation										
	b. Cer. Effacement										
	c. Membranes										
	d. Presentation Part										
	e. Station										
	f. Position of Occiput										
	PARAMETERS										
	q. FHS/min										
III.	r. Pulse/min										
	s. BP										
	t. Urine output										
IV.	**MEDICATION**										
V.	**SUPPORTIVE TREATMENT**										

IInd Stage

Membranes Ruptured at...AM/PM Spont/Artificial

Colour of Liqour...

Full Dilation /Explusive Cont Began at ....AM/PM On...

MOTHER:

Perineum: Rigid/Lax

Episiotomy: Given /Not Given

NEONATE:

Born at: ....AM/PM

On:..

Gender: Male/Female

Apgar Score 1min: ....

5 min: ....

Complication:

Treatment: Airway: ....

Eyes:..

Cord: ....

IIIrd Stage

a. Placenta and Membranes:

Delivered at .... AM/PM

Complete/Incomplete

Cord Insertion: Central/Marginal/Velamentous

Cord Length: .... (Inches)

Weight:...

b. Condition of Uterus:

c. PERINEUM: Episiotomy/Tear Laceration

Repair:...No.of Sutures ....No.of Catgut

d. Drugs given: ....

e. Approximate blood loss ....ml

PARTOGRAPH

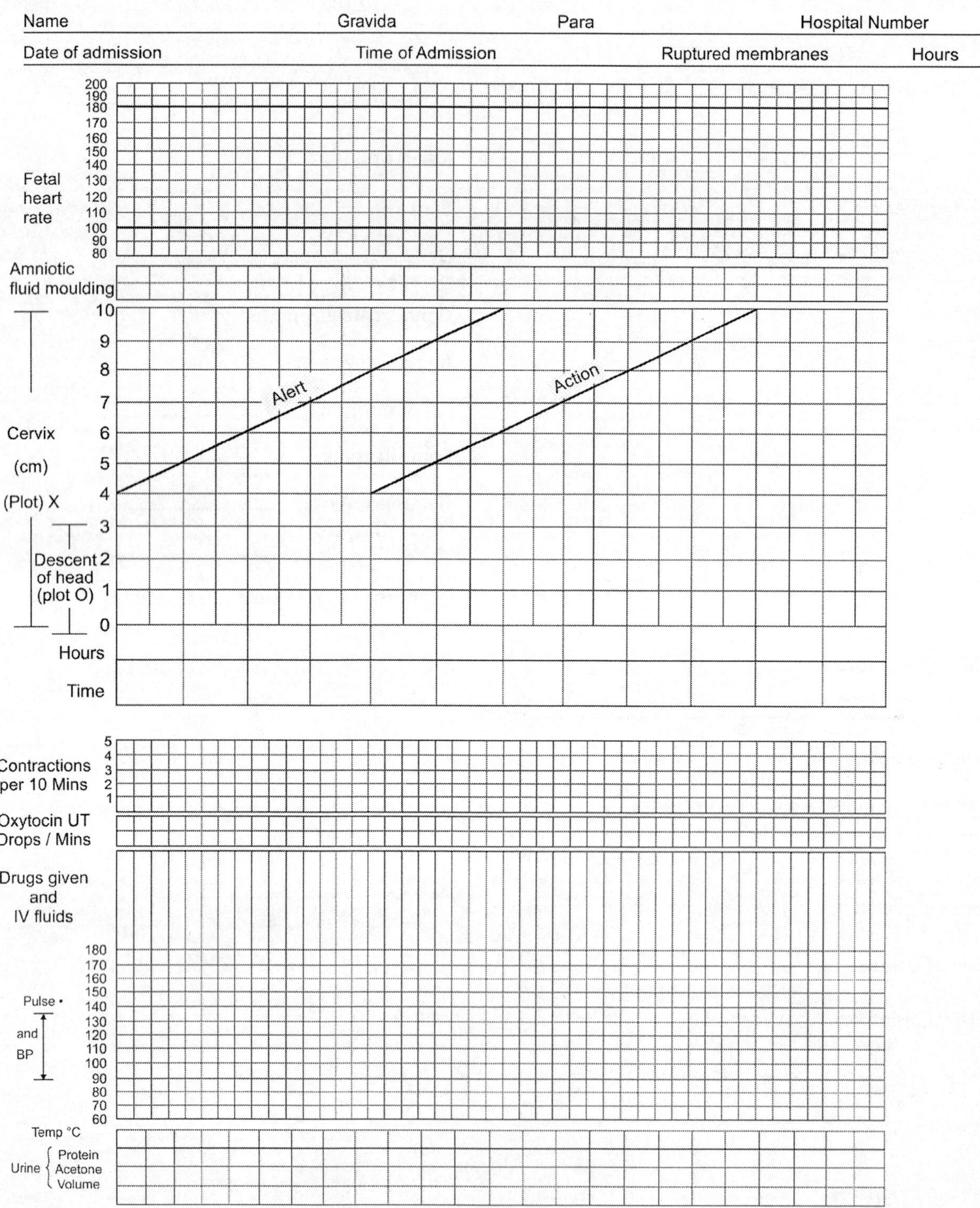

Name
Gravida
Para
Hospital Number
Date of admission
Time of Admission
Ruptured membranes
Hours
Fetal heart rate
200
190
180
170
160
150
140
130
120
110
100
90
80
Amniotic fluid moulding
Cervix (cm) (Plot) X
10
9
8
7
6
5
4
3
2
1
0
Alert
Action
Descent of head (plot O)
Hours
Time
Contractions per 10 Mins
5
4
3
2
1
Oxytocin UT Drops / Mins
Drugs given and IV fluids
Pulse •
and BP
180
170
160
150
140
130
120
110
100
90
80
70
60
Temp °C
Urine
Protein
Acetone
Volume

LABOUR SUMMARY

Type of labour: Spont/Induced

Mode of delivery: Vaginal/Instrument

Length of Labour:

1st stage .... Hrs .... Mins

2nd stage .... Hrs .... Mins

3rd stage .... Hrs .... Mins

Delivered by: ....

CONDUCTED CARE STUDY

IDENTIFICATION DATA

Name of the Mother:..

Reg.No:..

Age:..

Gravida:..

Parity:..

Date of Admission and Time:..

Date of Delivery and Time:..

Date of Discharge:..

PAST MENSTRUAL HISTORY

LMP ....EDD ....Cycle...

HEALTH HISTORY

1. Past Obstetrical History..

....

....

2. Present Pregnancy History

- I-trimester..

  ....

  ....

- II-trimester..

  ....

  ....

- III-trimester..

  ....

  ....

3. Past Medical History ....

....

....

4. Present Surgical History. ....

....

....

5. Past Surgical History. ....

....

....

6. Family History. ....

....

....

7. Personal History. ....

....

....

OBSTETRICAL HISTORY

S.No.	Year	Abortion	Prem	F.T.	Type of Labour and Mode of Delivery	Gender	Live or Still Birth	Remark

INVESTIGATION

USG Date: ....Finding: BPD..

FL/CRL..

Blood Group: .... Hb: .... Urine: ALB .... Placenta..

RH Factor: .... VDRL:...................................... Sug.................... .... Gest. Wks...

Liquor...

Anamoly..

ANTENATAL ATTENDANCES

LMP.............................. EDD...Gestation at 1st visit.................. wk

Date	Wt	BP	FHS	Weeks	Fundal height	Presentation	Treatments and Remarks

Labour Ward Admission Notes:

Admitted on:...at .... AM/PM

Contraction Commenced on: ....at .... AM/PM

Period of Gestation:...weeks

Height of Fundus...cms.

Presentation:...

Position: ....

Engaged /Not Engaged:

FHS:.. /min

Bladder: Voided/Catheter

Bowel: SE Given/Not Given (Reason)

Remarks if Any:...

LABOUR RECORD : 1st STAGE

I.	**OBSERVATION**										
	UTERINE CONTRATION										
	a. Frequency in 10 mins										
	b. Duration in Secs										
	c. Intensity										
II.	**PER VAGINAL EXAM**										
	a. Cervical Dilatation										
	b. Cer. Effacement										
	c. Membranes										
	d. Presentation Part										
	e. Station										
	f. Position of Occiput										
III.	**PARAMETERS**										
	u. FHS/min										
	v. Pulse/min										
	w. BP										
	x. Urine output										
IV.	**MEDICATION**										
V.	**SUPPORTIVE TREATMENT**										

IInd Stage

Membranes Ruptured at...AM/PM Spont/Artificial

Colour of Liqour...

Full Dilation /Explusive Cont Began at ....AM/PM On ....

MOTHER:

Perineum: Rigid/Lax

Episiotomy: Given /Not Given

NEONATE:

Born at: ....AM/PM

On:...

Gender: Male/Female

Apgar Score 1min:...

5 min: ....

Complication:

Treatment: Airway:..

Eyes:..

Cord:..

IIIrd Stage

a. Placenta and Membranes:

Delivered at.. AM/PM

Complete/Incomplete

Cord Insertion: Central/Marginal/Velamentous

Cord Length: .... (Inches)

Weight:...

b. Condition of Uterus:

c. PERINEUM: Episiotomy/Tear Laceration

Repair:...No.of Sutures ....No.of Catgut

d. Drugs given: ....

e. Approximate blood loss ....ml

PARTOGRAPH

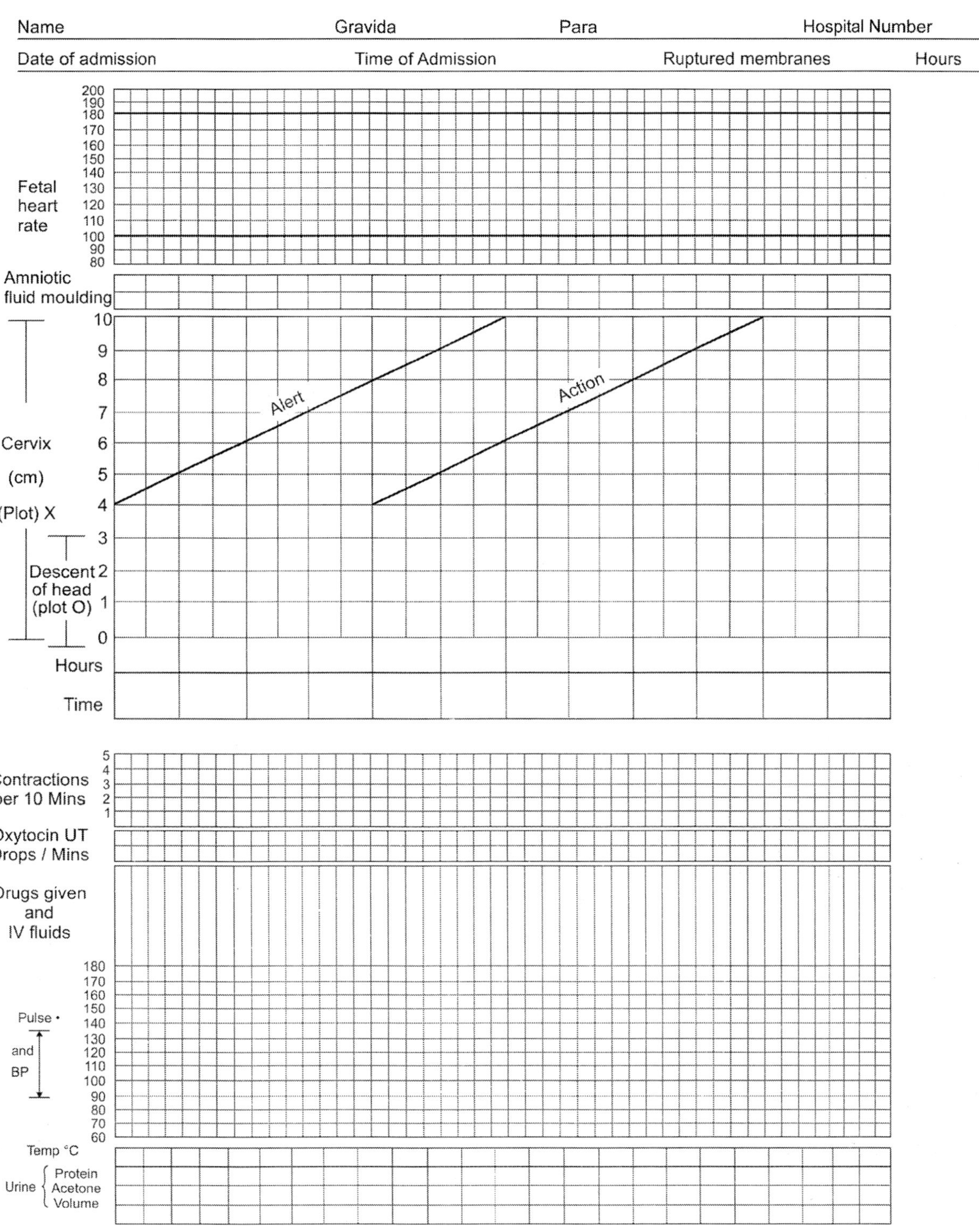

Name Gravida Para Hospital Number

Date of admission Time of Admission Ruptured membranes Hours

Fetal heart rate
200
190
180
170
160
150
140
130
120
110
100
90
80

Amniotic fluid moulding

Cervix (cm) (Plot) X
10
9
8
7
6
5
4
Alert
Action

Descent of head (plot O)
3
2
1
0

Hours

Time

Contractions per 10 Mins
5
4
3
2
1

Oxytocin UT Drops / Mins

Drugs given and IV fluids

Pulse •
and
BP
180
170
160
150
140
130
120
110
100
90
80
70
60

Temp °C

Urine
Protein
Acetone
Volume

LABOUR SUMMARY

Type of labour: Spont/Induced

Mode of delivery: Vaginal/Instrument

Length of Labour:

1st stage .... Hrs .... Mins

2nd stage .... Hrs .... Mins

3rd stage .... Hrs .... Mins

Delivered by: ....

CONDUCTED CARE STUDY

IDENTIFICATION DATA

Name of the Mother:...

Reg.No:...

Age:...

Gravida:...

Parity:...

Date of Admission and Time:...

Date of Delivery and Time:...

Date of Discharge:...

PAST MENSTRUAL HISTORY

LMP ....EDD ....Cycle..

HEALTH HISTORY

1. Past Obstetrical History...

....

....

2. Present Pregnancy History
   - I-trimester...

     ....

     ....
   - II-trimester...

     ....

     ....
   - III-trimester...

     ....

     ....

3. Past Medical History ....
....
....

4. Present Surgical History. ....
....
....

5. Past Surgical History. ....
....
....

6. Family History. ....
....
....

7. Personal History. ....
....
....

OBSTETRICAL HISTORY

S.No.	Year	Abortion	Prem	F.T.	Type of Labour and Mode of Delivery	Gender	Live or Still Birth	Remark

INVESTIGATION

USG Date: ....Finding: BPD...

FL/CRL..

Blood Group: .... Hb: .... Urine: ALB .... Placenta ....

RH Factor: .... VDRL:.................................... Sug................... .... Gest. Wks ....

Liquor ....

Anamoly ....

ANTENATAL ATTENDANCES							
LMP............................. EDD..Gestation at 1st visit.................. wk							
Date	Wt	BP	FHS	Weeks	Fundal height	Presentation	Treatments and Remarks

Labour Ward Admission Notes:

Admitted on:...at .... AM/PM

Contraction Commenced on: ....at .... AM/PM

Period of Gestation:...weeks

Height of Fundus ....cms.

Presentation:...

Position: ....

Engaged /Not Engaged:

FHS:... /min

Bladder: Voided/Catheter

Bowel: SE Given/Not Given (Reason)

Remarks if Any:..

LABOUR RECORD : 1st STAGE

I.	**OBSERVATION**										
	UTERINE CONTRATION										
	a. Frequency in 10 mins										
	b. Duration in Secs										
	c. Intensity										
II.	**PER VAGINAL EXAM**										
	a. Cervical Dilatation										
	b. Cer. Effacement										
	c. Membranes										
	d. Presentation Part										
	e. Station										
	f. Position of Occiput										
III.	**PARAMETERS**										
	y. FHS/min										
	z. Pulse/min										
	aa. BP										
	ab. Urine output										
IV.	**MEDICATION**										
V.	**SUPPORTIVE TREATMENT**										

IInd Stage

Membranes Ruptured at..AM/PM Spont/Artificial

Colour of Liqour..

Full Dilation /Explusive Cont Began at ....AM/PM On...

MOTHER:

Perineum: Rigid/Lax

Episiotomy: Given /Not Given

NEONATE:

Born at: ....AM/PM

On:...

Gender: Male/Female

Apgar Score 1min: ....

5 min: ....

Complication:

Treatment: Airway: ....

Eyes:..

Cord:...

IIIrd Stage

a. Placenta and Membranes:

Delivered at.. AM/PM

Complete/Incomplete

Cord Insertion: Central/Marginal/Velamentous

Cord Length: .... (Inches)

Weight:...

b. Condition of Uterus:

c. PERINEUM: Episiotomy/Tear Laceration

Repair:...No.of Sutures ....No.of Catgut

d. Drugs given: ....

e. Approximate blood loss ....ml

PARTOGRAPH

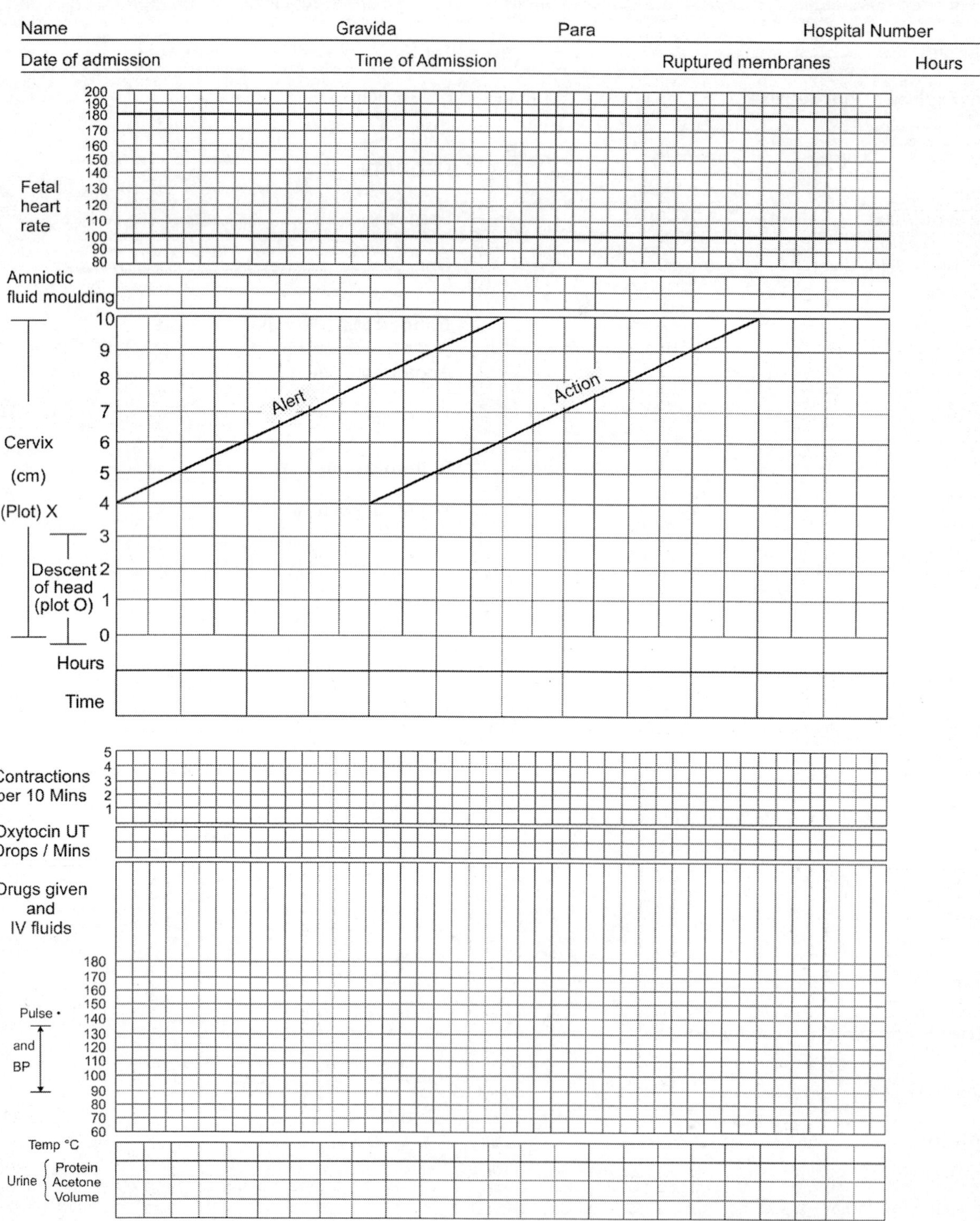
Name
Gravida
Para
Hospital Number
Date of admission
Time of Admission
Ruptured membranes
Hours
200
190
180
170
160
150
140
130
120
110
100
90
80
Fetal heart rate
Amniotic fluid moulding
10
9
8
7
6
5
4
3
2
1
0
Alert
Action
Cervix
(cm)
(Plot) X
Descent of head (plot O)
Hours
Time
Contractions per 10 Mins
5
4
3
2
1
Oxytocin UT Drops / Mins
Drugs given and IV fluids
Pulse •
and
BP
180
170
160
150
140
130
120
110
100
90
80
70
60
Temp °C
Urine
Protein
Acetone
Volume

LABOUR SUMMARY

Type of labour: Spont/Induced

Mode of delivery: Vaginal/Instrument

Length of Labour:

1st stage .... Hrs .... Mins

2nd stage .... Hrs .... Mins

3rd stage .... Hrs .... Mins

Delivered by: ....

CONDUCTED CARE STUDY

IDENTIFICATION DATA

Name of the Mother:...

Reg.No:...

Age:...

Gravida:...

Parity:..

Date of Admission and Time:...

Date of Delivery and Time:..

Date of Discharge:...

PAST MENSTRUAL HISTORY

LMP ....EDD ....Cycle...

HEALTH HISTORY

1. Past Obstetrical History...

   ....

   ....

2. Present Pregnancy History

   - I-trimester ....

     ....

     ....

   - II-trimester ....

     ....

     ....

   - III-trimester ....

     ....

     ....

3. Past Medical History ....

....

....

4. Present Surgical History. ....

....

....

5. Past Surgical History. ....

....

....

6. Family History. ....

....

....

7. Personal History. ....

....

....

OBSTETRICAL HISTORY

S.No.	Year	Abortion	Prem	F.T.	Type of Labour and Mode of Delivery	Gender	Live or Still Birth	Remark

INVESTIGATION

USG Date: ....Finding: BPD..

FL/CRL...

Blood Group: .... Hb: .... Urine: ALB .... Placenta..

RH Factor: .... VDRL:....................................... Sug.................... .... Gest. Wks..

Liquor...

Anamoly...

ANTENATAL ATTENDANCES

LMP.............................. EDD..Gestation at 1st visit.................. wk

Date	Wt	BP	FHS	Weeks	Fundal height	Presentation	Treatments and Remarks

Labour Ward Admission Notes:

Admitted on:..at .... AM/PM

Contraction Commenced on: ....at .... AM/PM

Period of Gestation:...weeks

Height of Fundus...cms.

Presentation:...

Position: ....

Engaged /Not Engaged:

FHS:... /min

Bladder: Voided/Catheter

Bowel: SE Given/Not Given (Reason)

Remarks if Any:...

LABOUR RECORD : 1st STAGE

I.	OBSERVATION										
	UTERINE CONTRATION										
	a. Frequency in 10 mins										
	b. Duration in Secs										
	c. Intensity										
II.	PER VAGINAL EXAM										
	a. Cervical Dilatation										
	b. Cer. Effacement										
	c. Membranes										
	d. Presentation Part										
	e. Station										
	f. Position of Occiput										
	PARAMETERS										
	ac. FHS/min										
III.	ad. Pulse/min										
	ae. BP										
	af. Urine output										
IV.	MEDICATION										
V.	SUPPORTIVE TREATMENT										

IInd Stage

Membranes Ruptured at..AM/PM Spont/Artificial

Colour of Liqour..

Full Dilation /Explusive Cont Began at ....AM/PM On..

MOTHER:

Perineum: Rigid/Lax

Episiotomy: Given /Not Given

NEONATE:

Born at: ....AM/PM

On:..

Gender: Male/Female

Apgar Score 1min:.......................................

5 min: ....

Complication:

Treatment: Airway:.......................................

Eyes:..

Cord:..

IIIrd Stage

a. Placenta and Membranes:

Delivered at... AM/PM

Complete/Incomplete

Cord Insertion: Central/Marginal/Velamentous

Cord Length: .... (Inches)

Weight:...

b. Condition of Uterus:

c. PERINEUM: Episiotomy/Tear Laceration

Repair:...No.of Sutures ....No.of Catgut

d. Drugs given: ....

e. Approximate blood loss ....ml

PARTOGRAPH

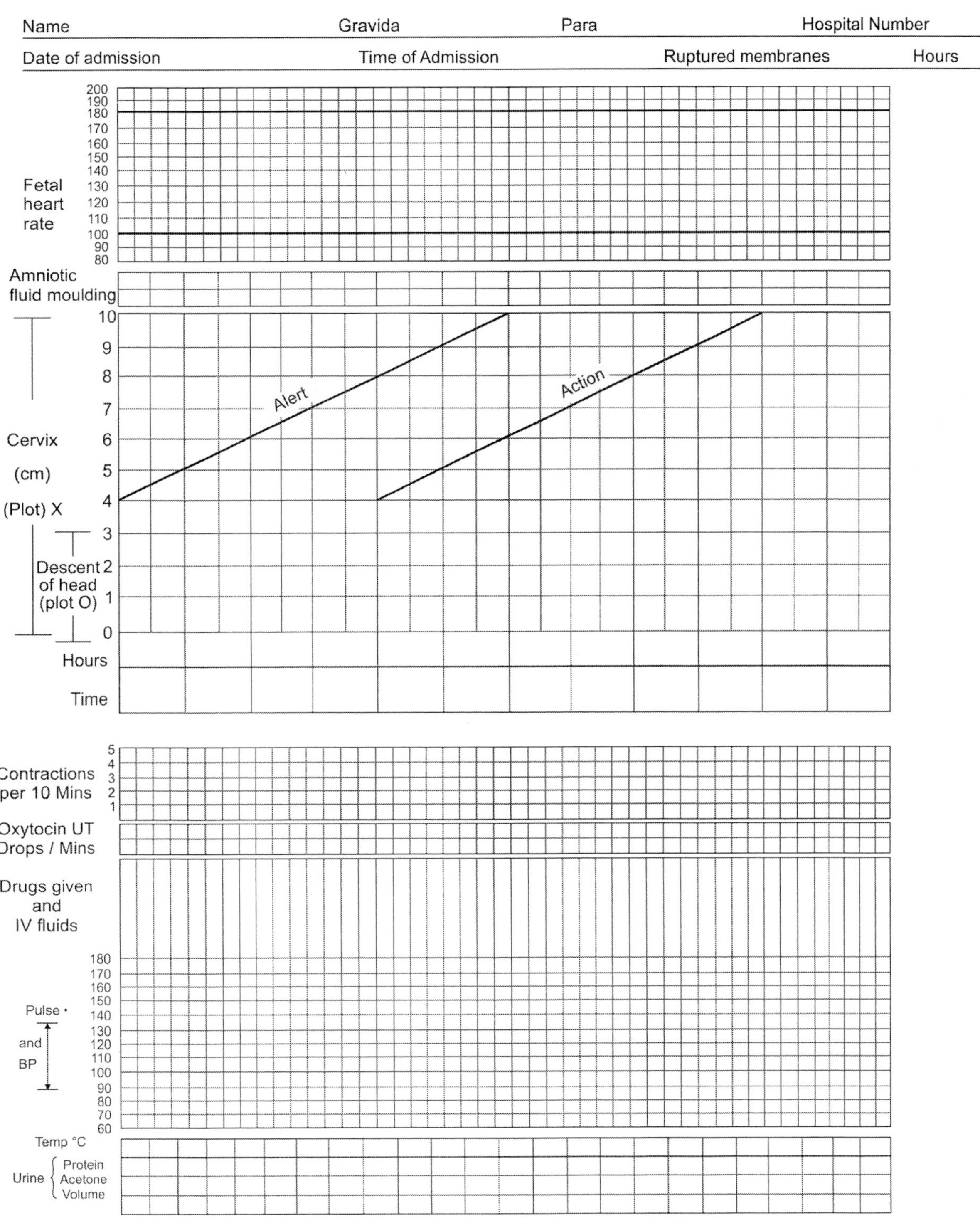
Name
Gravida
Para
Hospital Number
Date of admission
Time of Admission
Ruptured membranes
Hours
Fetal heart rate
200
190
180
170
160
150
140
130
120
110
100
90
80
Amniotic fluid moulding
Cervix (cm) (Plot) X
10
9
8
7
6
5
4
3
2
1
0
Alert
Action
Descent of head (plot O)
Hours
Time
Contractions per 10 Mins
5
4
3
2
1
Oxytocin UT Drops / Mins
Drugs given and IV fluids
Pulse •
and
BP
180
170
160
150
140
130
120
110
100
90
80
70
60
Temp °C
Urine
Protein
Acetone
Volume

LABOUR SUMMARY

Type of labour: Spont/Induced

Mode of delivery: Vaginal/Instrument

Length of Labour:

1st stage .... Hrs .... Mins

2nd stage .... Hrs .... Mins

3rd stage .... Hrs .... Mins

Delivered by: ....

CONDUCTED CARE STUDY

IDENTIFICATION DATA

Name of the Mother:..

Reg.No:..

Age:..

Gravida:..

Parity:..

Date of Admission and Time:..

Date of Delivery and Time:..

Date of Discharge:..

PAST MENSTRUAL HISTORY

LMP ....EDD ....Cycle...

HEALTH HISTORY

1. Past Obstetrical History..

   ....

   ....

2. Present Pregnancy History

   - I-trimester..

     ....

     ....

   - II-trimester..

     ....

     ....

   - III-trimester..

     ....

     ....

3. Past Medical History ....
....
....

4. Present Surgical History. ....
....
....

5. Past Surgical History. ....
....
....

6. Family History. ....
....
....

7. Personal History. ....
....
....

OBSTETRICAL HISTORY

S.No.	Year	Abortion	Prem	F.T.	Type of Labour and Mode of Delivery	Gender	Live or Still Birth	Remark

INVESTIGATION

USG Date: ....Finding: BPD...

FL/CRL..

Blood Group: .... Hb: .... Urine: ALB .... Placenta ....

RH Factor: .... VDRL:.................................... Sug.................. .... Gest. Wks ....

Liquor ....

Anamoly ....

ANTENATAL ATTENDANCES							
LMP............................ EDD...Gestation at 1st visit.................. wk							
Date	Wt	BP	FHS	Weeks	Fundal height	Presentation	Treatments and Remarks

Labour Ward Admission Notes:

Admitted on:.. at .... AM/PM

Contraction Commenced on: .... at .... AM/PM

Period of Gestation:.. weeks

Height of Fundus .... cms.

Presentation: ....

Position: ....

Engaged /Not Engaged:

FHS:.. /min

Bladder: Voided/Catheter

Bowel: SE Given/Not Given (Reason)

Remarks if Any:...

LABOUR RECORD : 1st STAGE

I.	**OBSERVATION**										
	UTERINE CONTRATION										
	a. Frequency in 10 mins										
	b. Duration in Secs										
	c. Intensity										
II.	**PER VAGINAL EXAM**										
	a. Cervical Dilatation										
	b. Cer. Effacement										
	c. Membranes										
	d. Presentation Part										
	e. Station										
	f. Position of Occiput										
	PARAMETERS										
	ag. FHS/min										
III.	ah. Pulse/min										
	ai. BP										
	aj. Urine output										
IV.	**MEDICATION**										
V.	**SUPPORTIVE TREATMENT**										

IInd Stage

Membranes Ruptured at...AM/PM Spont/Artificial

Colour of Liqour..

Full Dilation /Explusive Cont Began at ....AM/PM On...

MOTHER:

Perineum: Rigid/Lax

Episiotomy: Given /Not Given

NEONATE:

Born at: .... AM/PM

On:...

Gender: Male/Female

Apgar Score 1min: ....

5 min: ....

Complication:

Treatment: Airway: ....

Eyes:...

Cord: ....

IIIrd Stage

a. Placenta and Membranes:

Delivered at .... AM/PM

Complete/Incomplete

Cord Insertion: Central/Marginal/Velamentous

Cord Length: .... (Inches)

Weight:..

b. Condition of Uterus:

c. PERINEUM: Episiotomy/Tear Laceration

Repair:...No.of Sutures ....No.of Catgut

d. Drugs given: ....

e. Approximate blood loss ....ml

PARTOGRAPH

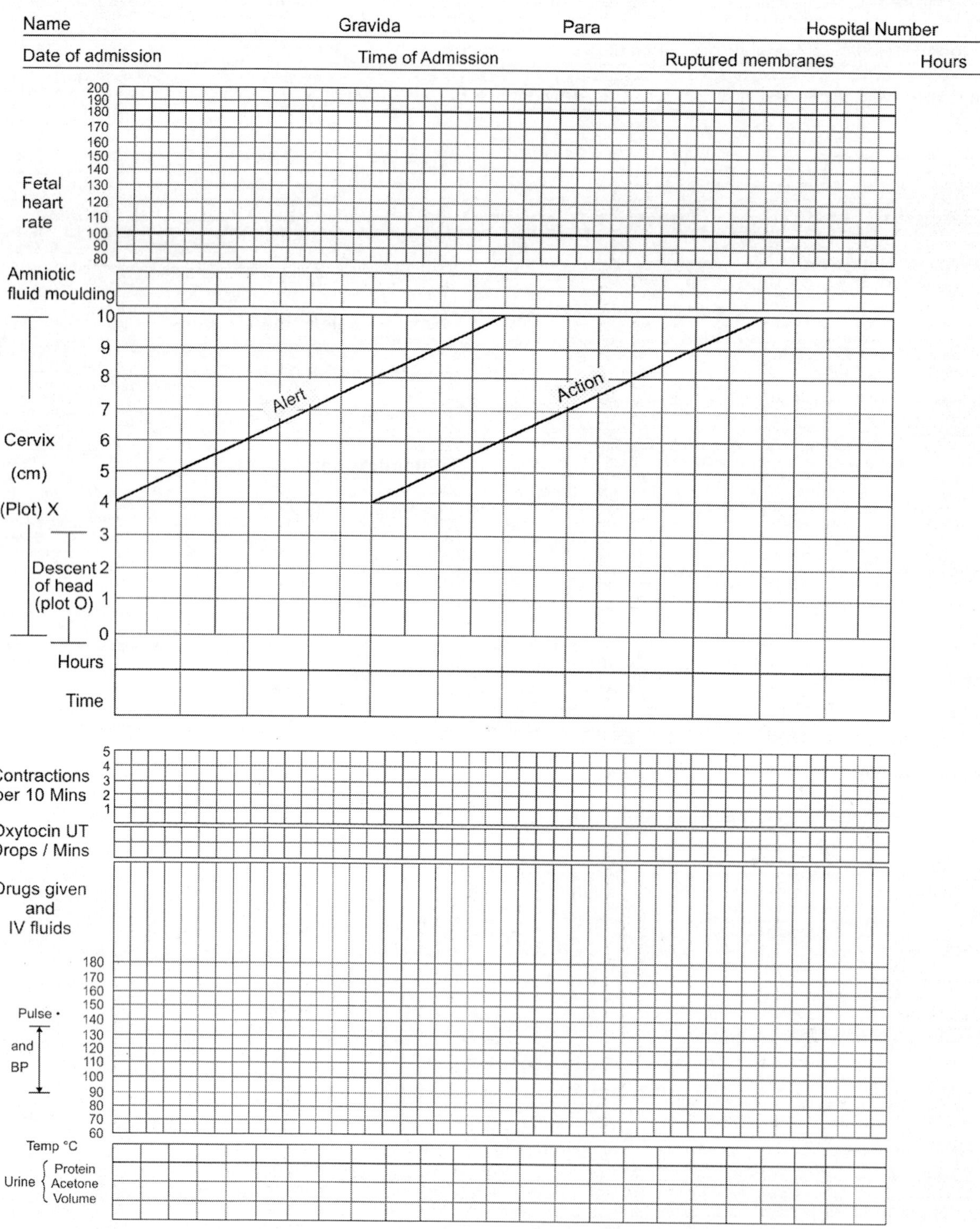
Name
Gravida
Para
Hospital Number
Date of admission
Time of Admission
Ruptured membranes
Hours
Fetal heart rate
200
190
180
170
160
150
140
130
120
110
100
90
80
Amniotic fluid moulding
10
9
8
7
6
5
4
3
2
1
0
Alert
Action
Cervix (cm) (Plot) X
Descent of head (plot O)
Hours
Time
Contractions per 10 Mins
5
4
3
2
1
Oxytocin UT Drops / Mins
Drugs given and IV fluids
Pulse •
and BP
180
170
160
150
140
130
120
110
100
90
80
70
60
Temp °C
Urine
Protein
Acetone
Volume

LABOUR SUMMARY

Type of labour: Spont/Induced

Mode of delivery: Vaginal/Instrument

Length of Labour:

1st stage .... Hrs .... Mins

2nd stage .... Hrs .... Mins

3rd stage .... Hrs .... Mins

Delivered by: ....

CONDUCTED CARE STUDY

IDENTIFICATION DATA

Name of the Mother:..

Reg.No: ....

Age:..

Gravida: ....

Parity: ....

Date of Admission and Time: ....

Date of Delivery and Time:..

Date of Discharge:..

PAST MENSTRUAL HISTORY

LMP ....EDD ....Cycle..

HEALTH HISTORY

1. Past Obstetrical History..

   ....

   ....

2. Present Pregnancy History

   - I-trimester ....

     ....

     ....

   - II-trimester ....

     ....

     ....

   - III-trimester..

     ....

     ....

3. Past Medical History ....

....

....

4. Present Surgical History. ....

....

....

5. Past Surgical History. ....

....

....

6. Family History. ....

....

....

7. Personal History. ....

....

....

OBSTETRICAL HISTORY

S.No.	Year	Abortion	Prem	F.T.	Type of Labour and Mode of Delivery	Gender	Live or Still Birth	Remark

INVESTIGATION

USG Date: ....Finding: BPD...

FL/CRL...

Blood Group: .... Hb: .... Urine: ALB .... Placenta ....

RH Factor: .... VDRL:....................................... Sug.................... .... Gest. Wks ....

Liquor ....

Anamoly ....

ANTENATAL ATTENDANCES

LMP............................. EDD..Gestation at 1st visit.................. wk

Date	Wt	BP	FHS	Weeks	Fundal height	Presentation	Treatments and Remarks

Labour Ward Admission Notes:

Admitted on:...at .... AM/PM

Contraction Commenced on: ....at .... AM/PM

Period of Gestation:...weeks

Height of Fundus ....cms.

Presentation: ....

Position: ....

Engaged /Not Engaged:

FHS:... /min

Bladder: Voided/Catheter

Bowel: SE Given/Not Given (Reason)

Remarks if Any:...

LABOUR RECORD : 1st STAGE

I.	**OBSERVATION**										
	UTERINE CONTRATION										
	a. Frequency in 10 mins										
	b. Duration in Secs										
	c. Intensity										
II.	**PER VAGINAL EXAM**										
	a. Cervical Dilatation										
	b. Cer. Effacement										
	c. Membranes										
	d. Presentation Part										
	e. Station										
	f. Position of Occiput										
	PARAMETERS										
	ak. FHS/min										
III.	al. Pulse/min										
	am. BP										
	an. Urine output										
IV.	**MEDICATION**										
V.	**SUPPORTIVE TREATMENT**										

IInd Stage

Membranes Ruptured at..AM/PM Spont/Artificial

Colour of Liqour..

Full Dilation /Explusive Cont Began at ....AM/PM On...

MOTHER:

Perineum: Rigid/Lax

Episiotomy: Given /Not Given

NEONATE:

Born at: ....AM/PM

On:...

Gender: Male/Female

Apgar Score 1min:..

5 min: ....

Complication:

Treatment: Airway:.......................................

Eyes:..

Cord:..

IIIrd Stage

a. Placenta and Membranes:

Delivered at .... AM/PM

Complete/Incomplete

Cord Insertion: Central/Marginal/Velamentous

Cord Length: .... (Inches)

Weight:..

b. Condition of Uterus:

c. PERINEUM: Episiotomy/Tear Laceration

Repair:...No.of Sutures ....No.of Catgut

d. Drugs given: ....

e. Approximate blood loss ....ml

PARTOGRAPH

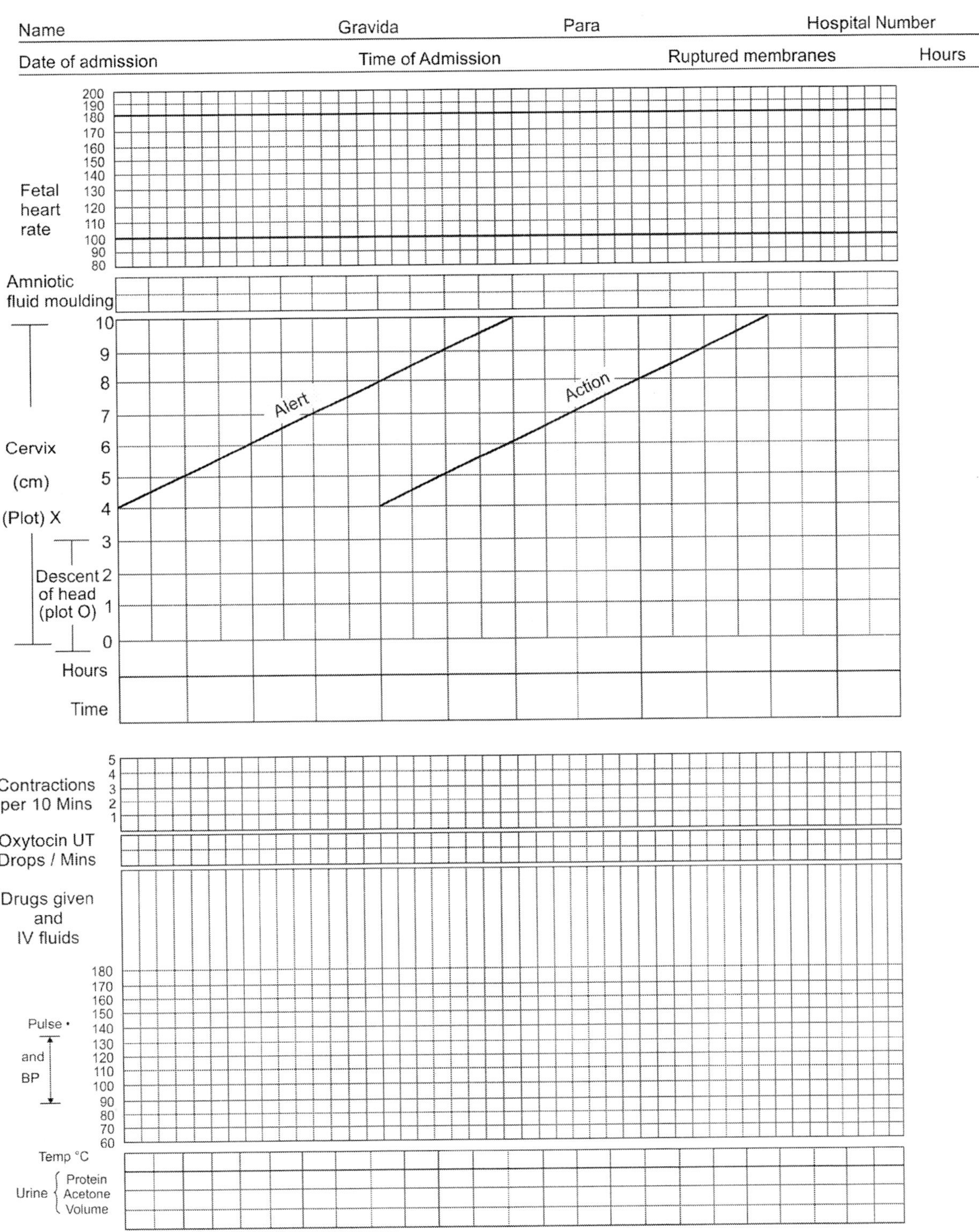

Name
Gravida
Para
Hospital Number
Date of admission
Time of Admission
Ruptured membranes
Hours
Fetal heart rate
200
190
180
170
160
150
140
130
120
110
100
90
80
Amniotic fluid moulding
Cervix (cm) (Plot) X
10
9
8
7
6
5
4
3
2
1
0
Alert
Action
Descent of head (plot O)
Hours
Time
Contractions per 10 Mins
5
4
3
2
1
Oxytocin UT Drops / Mins
Drugs given and IV fluids
Pulse •
and
BP
180
170
160
150
140
130
120
110
100
90
80
70
60
Temp °C
Urine
Protein
Acetone
Volume

LABOUR SUMMARY

Type of labour: Spont/Induced

Mode of delivery: Vaginal/Instrument

Length of Labour:

1st stage .... Hrs .... Mins

2nd stage .... Hrs .... Mins

3rd stage .... Hrs .... Mins

Delivered by: ....

CONDUCTED CARE STUDY

IDENTIFICATION DATA

Name of the Mother:..

Reg.No:..

Age:..

Gravida:..

Parity:..

Date of Admission and Time:..

Date of Delivery and Time:..

Date of Discharge:..

PAST MENSTRUAL HISTORY

LMP ....EDD ....Cycle..

HEALTH HISTORY

1. Past Obstetrical History..

....

....

2. Present Pregnancy History
   - I-trimester..

     ....

     ....
   - II-trimester..

     ....

     ....
   - III-trimester..

     ....

     ....

3. Past Medical History ....

....

....

4. Present Surgical History. ....

....

....

5. Past Surgical History. ....

....

....

6. Family History. ....

....

....

7. Personal History. ....

....

....

OBSTETRICAL HISTORY

S.No.	Year	Abortion	Prem	F.T.	Type of Labour and Mode of Delivery	Gender	Live or Still Birth	Remark

INVESTIGATION

USG Date: ....Finding: BPD..

FL/CRL..

Blood Group: .... Hb: .... Urine: ALB .... Placenta ....

RH Factor: .... VDRL:.................................... Sug.................... .... Gest. Wks ....

Liquor ....

Anamoly ....

ANTENATAL ATTENDANCES							
LMP............................ EDD...Gestation at 1st visit.................. wk							
Date	Wt	BP	FHS	Weeks	Fundal height	Presentation	Treatments and Remarks

Labour Ward Admission Notes:

Admitted on:.. at .... AM/PM

Contraction Commenced on: ....at .... AM/PM

Period of Gestation:...weeks

Height of Fundus...cms.

Presentation:..

Position: ....

Engaged /Not Engaged:

FHS:... /min

Bladder: Voided/Catheter

Bowel: SE Given/Not Given (Reason)

Remarks if Any:...

LABOUR RECORD : 1st STAGE											
I.	**OBSERVATION**										
	UTERINE CONTRATION										
	a. Frequency in 10 mins										
	b. Duration in Secs										
	c. Intensity										
II.	**PER VAGINAL EXAM**										
	a. Cervical Dilatation										
	b. Cer. Effacement										
	c. Membranes										
	d. Presentation Part										
	e. Station										
	f. Position of Occiput										
III.	**PARAMETERS**										
	ao. FHS/min										
	ap. Pulse/min										
	aq. BP										
	ar. Urine output										
IV.	**MEDICATION**										
V.	**SUPPORTIVE TREATMENT**										

IInd Stage

Membranes Ruptured at..AM/PM Spont/Artificial

Colour of Liqour..

Full Dilation /Explusive Cont Began at ....AM/PM On ....

MOTHER:

Perineum: Rigid/Lax

Episiotomy: Given /Not Given

NEONATE:

Born at: ....AM/PM

On:..

Gender: Male/Female

Apgar Score 1min:..

5 min: ....

Complication:

Treatment: Airway:..

Eyes:..

Cord:..

IIIrd Stage

a. Placenta and Membranes:

Delivered at.. AM/PM

Complete/Incomplete

Cord Insertion: Central/Marginal/Velamentous

Cord Length: .... (Inches)

Weight:...

b. Condition of Uterus:

c. PERINEUM: Episiotomy/Tear Laceration

Repair:...No.of Sutures ....No.of Catgut

d. Drugs given: ....

e. Approximate blood loss ....ml

PARTOGRAPH

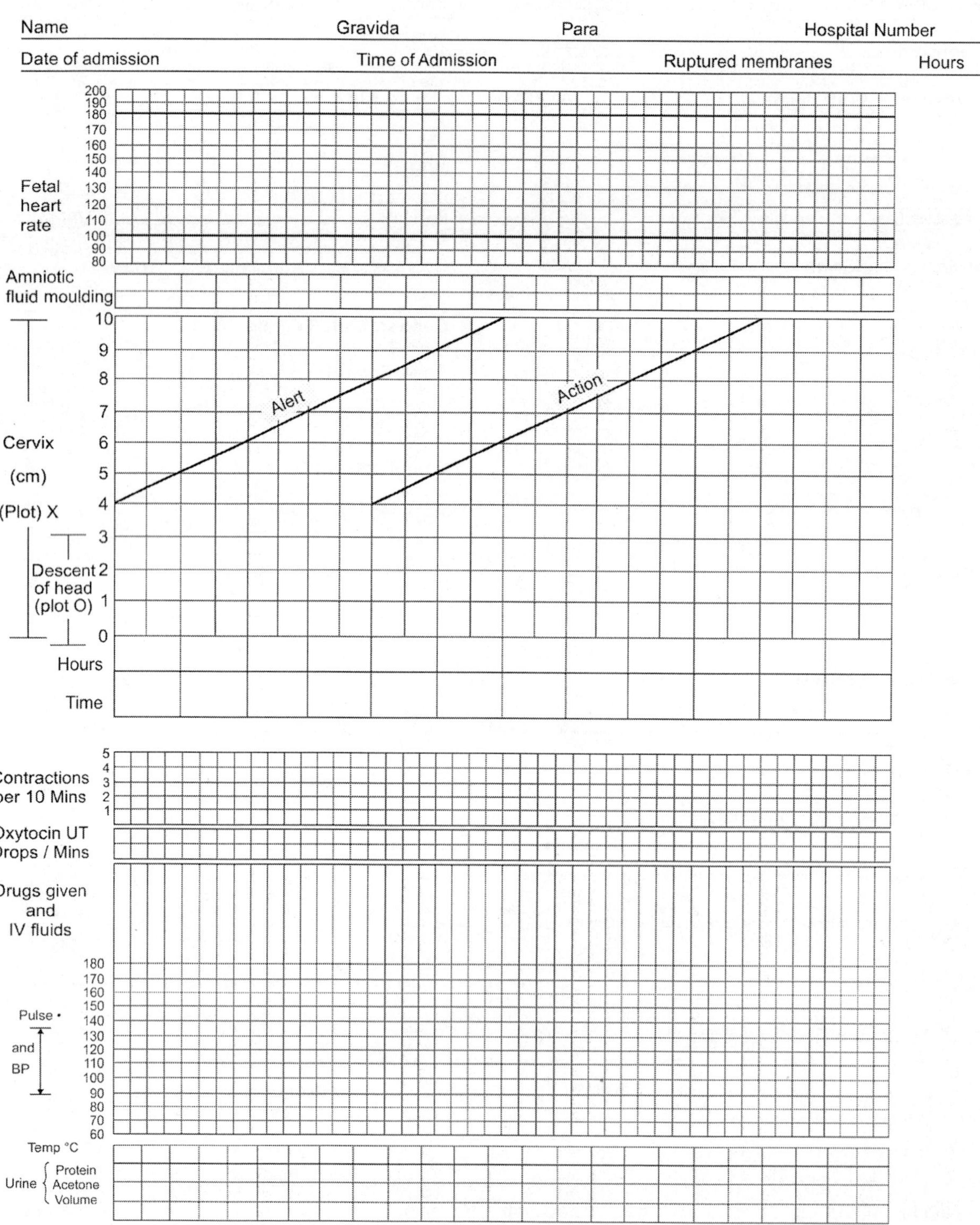
Name
Gravida
Para
Hospital Number
Date of admission
Time of Admission
Ruptured membranes
Hours
Fetal heart rate
200
190
180
170
160
150
140
130
120
110
100
90
80
Amniotic fluid moulding
Cervix (cm) (Plot) X
10
9
8
7
6
5
4
3
2
1
0
Alert
Action
Descent of head (plot O)
Hours
Time
Contractions per 10 Mins
5
4
3
2
1
Oxytocin UT Drops / Mins
Drugs given and IV fluids
Pulse •
and BP
180
170
160
150
140
130
120
110
100
90
80
70
60
Temp °C
Urine
Protein
Acetone
Volume

LABOUR SUMMARY

Type of labour: Spont/Induced

Mode of delivery: Vaginal/Instrument

Length of Labour:

1st stage .... Hrs .... Mins

2nd stage .... Hrs .... Mins

3rd stage .... Hrs .... Mins

Delivered by: ....

CONDUCTED CARE STUDY

IDENTIFICATION DATA

Name of the Mother:..

Reg.No:..

Age:..

Gravida:..

Parity:..

Date of Admission and Time:..

Date of Delivery and Time:..

Date of Discharge:..

PAST MENSTRUAL HISTORY

LMP .... EDD .... Cycle ....

HEALTH HISTORY

1. Past Obstetrical History..

   ....

   ....

2. Present Pregnancy History

   - I-trimester..

     ....

     ....

   - II-trimester..

     ....

     ....

   - III-trimester..

     ....

     ....

3. Past Medical History ....

....

....

4. Present Surgical History. ....

....

....

5. Past Surgical History. ....

....

....

6. Family History. ....

....

....

7. Personal History. ....

....

....

OBSTETRICAL HISTORY

S.No.	Year	Abortion	Prem	F.T.	Type of Labour and Mode of Delivery	Gender	Live or Still Birth	Remark

INVESTIGATION

USG Date: ....Finding: BPD..

FL/CRL...

Blood Group: .... Hb: .... Urine: ALB .... Placenta ....

RH Factor: .... VDRL:.................................... Sug.................. .... Gest. Wks ....

Liquor ....

Anamoly ....

ANTENATAL ATTENDANCES							
LMP............................ EDD..Gestation at 1st visit.................. wk							
Date	Wt	BP	FHS	Weeks	Fundal height	Presentation	Treatments and Remarks

Labour Ward Admission Notes:

Admitted on:..at .... AM/PM

Contraction Commenced on: ....at .... AM/PM

Period of Gestation:...weeks

Height of Fundus ....cms.

Presentation:..

Position: ....

Engaged /Not Engaged:

FHS:.. /min

Bladder: Voided/Catheter

Bowel: SE Given/Not Given (Reason)

Remarks if Any:..

LABOUR RECORD : 1st STAGE											
I.	**OBSERVATION**										
	UTERINE CONTRATION										
	a. Frequency in 10 mins										
	b. Duration in Secs										
	c. Intensity										
II.	**PER VAGINAL EXAM**										
	a. Cervical Dilatation										
	b. Cer. Effacement										
	c. Membranes										
	d. Presentation Part										
	e. Station										
	f. Position of Occiput										
III.	**PARAMETERS**										
	as. FHS/min										
	at. Pulse/min										
	au. BP										
	av. Urine output										
IV.	**MEDICATION**										
V.	**SUPPORTIVE TREATMENT**										

IInd Stage

Membranes Ruptured at..AM/PM Spont/Artificial

Colour of Liqour...

Full Dilation /Explusive Cont Began at ....AM/PM On..

MOTHER:

Perineum: Rigid/Lax

Episiotomy: Given /Not Given

NEONATE:

Born at: ....AM/PM

On:...

Gender: Male/Female

Apgar Score 1min: ....

5 min: ....

Complication:

Treatment: Airway: ....

Eyes:..

Cord: ....

IIIrd Stage

a. Placenta and Membranes:

Delivered at .... AM/PM

Complete/Incomplete

Cord Insertion: Central/Marginal/Velamentous

Cord Length: .... (Inches)

Weight:...

b. Condition of Uterus:

c. PERINEUM: Episiotomy/Tear Laceration

Repair:..No.of Sutures ....No.of Catgut

d. Drugs given: ....

e. Approximate blood loss ....ml

PARTOGRAPH

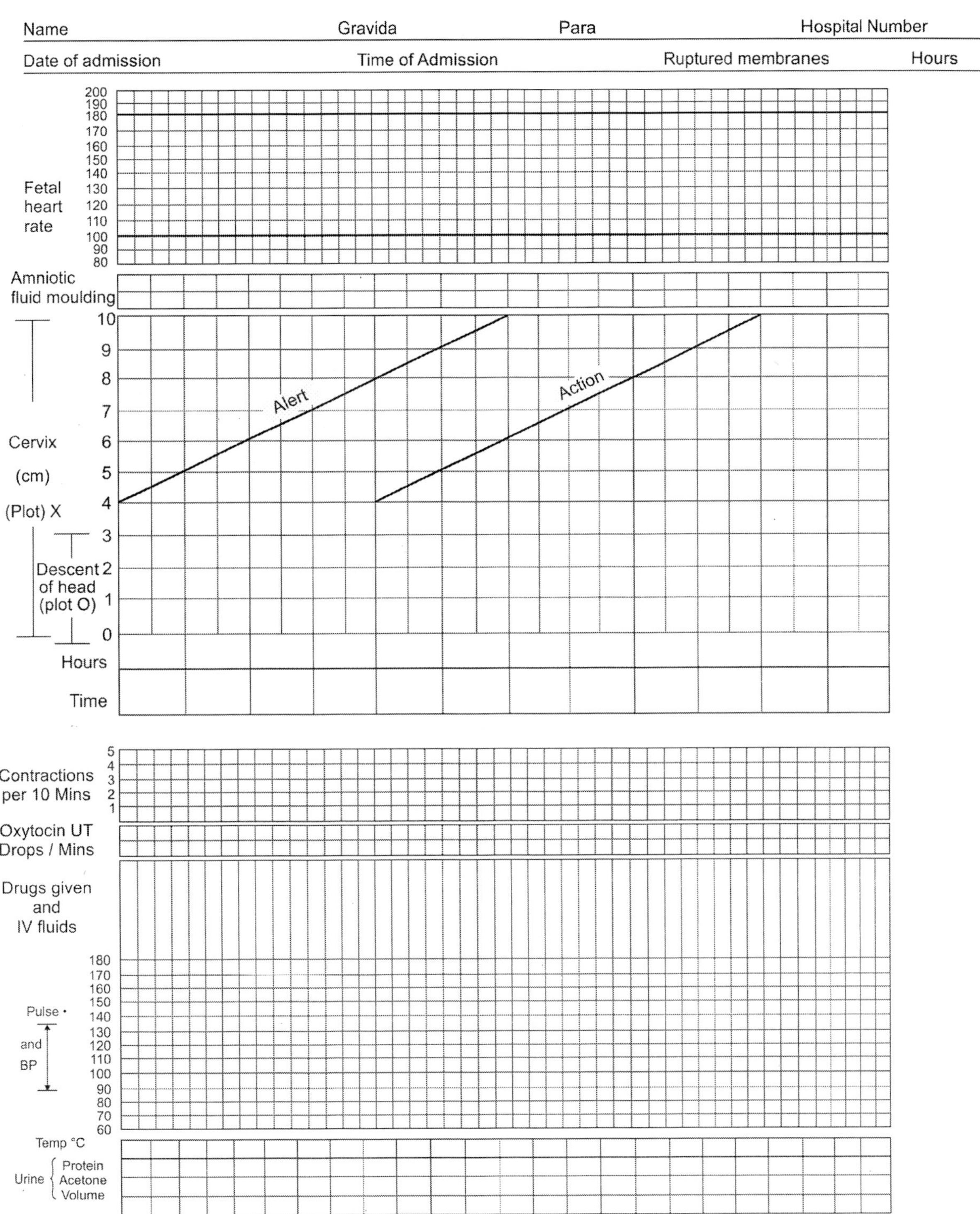
Name
Gravida
Para
Hospital Number
Date of admission
Time of Admission
Ruptured membranes
Hours
Fetal heart rate
200
190
180
170
160
150
140
130
120
110
100
90
80
Amniotic fluid moulding
Cervix (cm) (Plot) X
10
9
8
7
6
5
4
3
2
1
0
Alert
Action
Descent of head (plot O)
Hours
Time
Contractions per 10 Mins
5
4
3
2
1
Oxytocin UT Drops / Mins
Drugs given and IV fluids
Pulse •
and BP
180
170
160
150
140
130
120
110
100
90
80
70
60
Temp °C
Urine
Protein
Acetone
Volume

LABOUR SUMMARY

Type of labour: Spont/Induced

Mode of delivery: Vaginal/Instrument

Length of Labour:

1st stage .... Hrs .... Mins

2nd stage .... Hrs .... Mins

3rd stage .... Hrs .... Mins

Delivered by: ....

CONDUCTED CARE STUDY

IDENTIFICATION DATA

Name of the Mother:..

Reg.No:..

Age:..

Gravida:..

Parity:..

Date of Admission and Time: ....

Date of Delivery and Time:..

Date of Discharge:..

PAST MENSTRUAL HISTORY

LMP ....EDD ....Cycle..

HEALTH HISTORY

1. Past Obstetrical History..

   ....

   ....

2. Present Pregnancy History

   - I-trimester ....

     ....

     ....

   - II-trimester..

     ....

     ....

   - III-trimester..

     ....

     ....

3. Past Medical History ....
....
....

4. Present Surgical History. ....
....
....

5. Past Surgical History. ....
....
....

6. Family History. ....
....
....

7. Personal History. ....
....
....

OBSTETRICAL HISTORY

S.No.	Year	Abortion	Prem	F.T.	Type of Labour and Mode of Delivery	Gender	Live or Still Birth	Remark

INVESTIGATION

USG Date: ....Finding: BPD..

FL/CRL...

Blood Group: .... Hb: .... Urine: ALB...................... Placenta..

RH Factor: .... VDRL:...................................... Sug.................. .... Gest. Wks..

Liquor..

Anamoly..

ANTENATAL ATTENDANCES

LMP............................. EDD...Gestation at 1st visit.................. wk

Date	Wt	BP	FHS	Weeks	Fundal height	Presentation	Treatments and Remarks

Labour Ward Admission Notes:

Admitted on:...at .... AM/PM

Contraction Commenced on: ....at .... AM/PM

Period of Gestation:...weeks

Height of Fundus..cms.

Presentation:...

Position: ....

Engaged /Not Engaged:

FHS:... /min

Bladder: Voided/Catheter

Bowel: SE Given/Not Given (Reason)

Remarks if Any:...

LABOUR RECORD : 1st STAGE

I.	**OBSERVATION**										
	UTERINE CONTRATION										
	a. Frequency in 10 mins										
	b. Duration in Secs										
	c. Intensity										
II.	**PER VAGINAL EXAM**										
	a. Cervical Dilatation										
	b. Cer. Effacement										
	c. Membranes										
	d. Presentation Part										
	e. Station										
	f. Position of Occiput										
	PARAMETERS										
	aw. FHS/min										
III.	ax. Pulse/min										
	ay. BP										
	az. Urine output										
IV.	**MEDICATION**										
V.	**SUPPORTIVE TREATMENT**										

IInd Stage

Membranes Ruptured at...AM/PM Spont/Artificial

Colour of Liqour..

Full Dilation /Explusive Cont Began at ....AM/PM On..

MOTHER:

Perineum: Rigid/Lax

Episiotomy: Given /Not Given

NEONATE:

Born at: ....AM/PM

On:..

Gender: Male/Female

Apgar Score 1min:..

5 min: ....

Complication:

Treatment: Airway:.......................................

Eyes:...

Cord:..

IIIrd Stage

a. Placenta and Membranes:

Delivered at... AM/PM

Complete/Incomplete

Cord Insertion: Central/Marginal/Velamentous

Cord Length: .... (Inches)

Weight:...

b. Condition of Uterus:

c. PERINEUM: Episiotomy/Tear Laceration

Repair:..No.of Sutures ....No.of Catgut

d. Drugs given: ....

e. Approximate blood loss ....ml

PARTOGRAPH

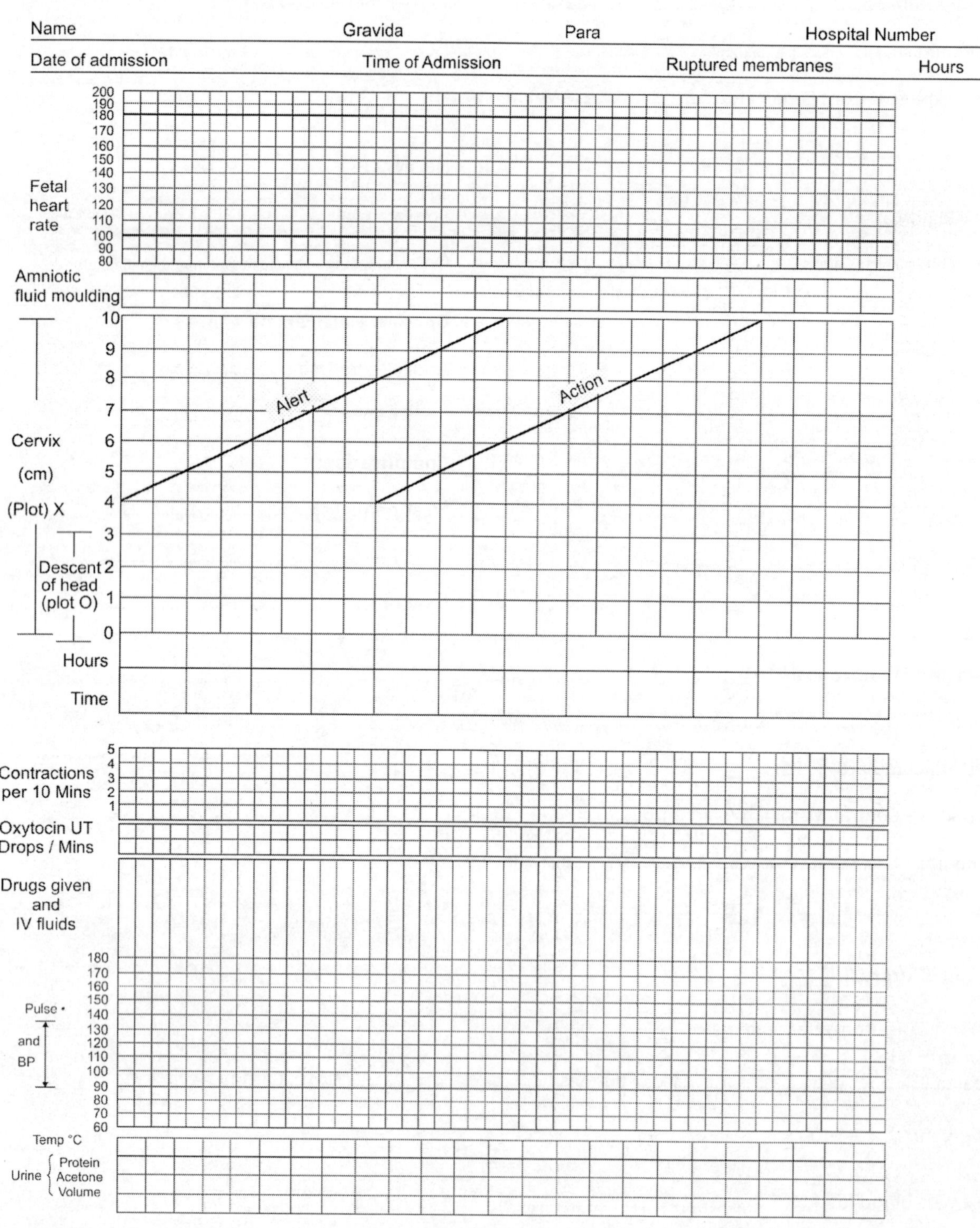
Name
Gravida
Para
Hospital Number
Date of admission
Time of Admission
Ruptured membranes
Hours
Fetal heart rate
200
190
180
170
160
150
140
130
120
110
100
90
80
Amniotic fluid moulding
Cervix (cm) (Plot) X
10
9
8
7
6
5
4
3
2
1
0
Alert
Action
Descent of head (plot O)
Hours
Time
Contractions per 10 Mins
5
4
3
2
1
Oxytocin UT Drops / Mins
Drugs given and IV fluids
Pulse •
and
BP
180
170
160
150
140
130
120
110
100
90
80
70
60
Temp °C
Urine
Protein
Acetone
Volume

LABOUR SUMMARY

Type of labour: Spont/Induced

Mode of delivery: Vaginal/Instrument

Length of Labour:

1st stage .... Hrs .... Mins

2nd stage .... Hrs .... Mins

3rd stage.. Hrs .... Mins

Delivered by: ....

CONDUCTED CARE STUDY

IDENTIFICATION DATA

Name of the Mother:..

Reg.No:..

Age:..

Gravida:..

Parity:..

Date of Admission and Time: ....

Date of Delivery and Time:..

Date of Discharge:..

PAST MENSTRUAL HISTORY

LMP ....EDD ....Cycle..............................

HEALTH HISTORY

1. Past Obstetrical History..

....

....

2. Present Pregnancy History

- I-trimester ....

  ....

  ....

- II-trimester..

  ....

  ....

- III-trimester..

  ....

  ....

3. Past Medical History ....

....

....

4. Present Surgical History. ....

....

....

5. Past Surgical History. ....

....

....

6. Family History. ....

....

....

7. Personal History. ....

....

....

OBSTETRICAL HISTORY

S.No.	Year	Abortion	Prem	F.T.	Type of Labour and Mode of Delivery	Gender	Live or Still Birth	Remark

INVESTIGATION

USG Date: ....Finding: BPD...

FL/CRL..

Blood Group: .... Hb: .... Urine: ALB .... Placenta..

RH Factor: .... VDRL:.................................... Sug.................... .... Gest. Wks...

Liquor ....

Anamoly...

ANTENATAL ATTENDANCES

LMP............................. EDD..Gestation at 1st visit.................. wk

Date	Wt	BP	FHS	Weeks	Fundal height	Presentation	Treatments and Remarks

Labour Ward Admission Notes:

Admitted on:.. at .... AM/PM

Contraction Commenced on: .... at .... AM/PM

Period of Gestation:.. weeks

Height of Fundus... cms.

Presentation:..

Position: ....

Engaged /Not Engaged:

FHS:.. /min

Bladder: Voided/Catheter

Bowel: SE Given/Not Given (Reason)

Remarks if Any:...

LABOUR RECORD : 1st STAGE

I.	**OBSERVATION**										
	UTERINE CONTRATION										
	a. Frequency in 10 mins										
	b. Duration in Secs										
	c. Intensity										
II.	**PER VAGINAL EXAM**										
	a. Cervical Dilatation										
	b. Cer. Effacement										
	c. Membranes										
	d. Presentation Part										
	e. Station										
	f. Position of Occiput										
	PARAMETERS										
	ba. FHS/min										
III.	bb. Pulse/min										
	bc. BP										
	bd. Urine output										
IV.	**MEDICATION**										
V.	**SUPPORTIVE TREATMENT**										

IInd Stage

Membranes Ruptured at...AM/PM Spont/Artificial

Colour of Liqour...

Full Dilation /Explusive Cont Began at ....AM/PM On...

MOTHER:

Perineum: Rigid/Lax

Episiotomy: Given /Not Given

NEONATE:

Born at: ....AM/PM

On:..

Gender: Male/Female

Apgar Score 1min: ....

5 min: ....

Complication:

Treatment: Airway: ....

Eyes: ....

Cord: ....

IIIrd Stage

a. **Placenta and Membranes:**

Delivered at... AM/PM

Complete/Incomplete

Cord Insertion: Central/Marginal/Velamentous

Cord Length: .... (Inches)

Weight:...

b. **Condition of Uterus:**

c. **PERINEUM:** Episiotomy/Tear Laceration

Repair:...No.of Sutures ....No.of Catgut

d. **Drugs given:** ....

e. Approximate blood loss ....ml

PARTOGRAPH

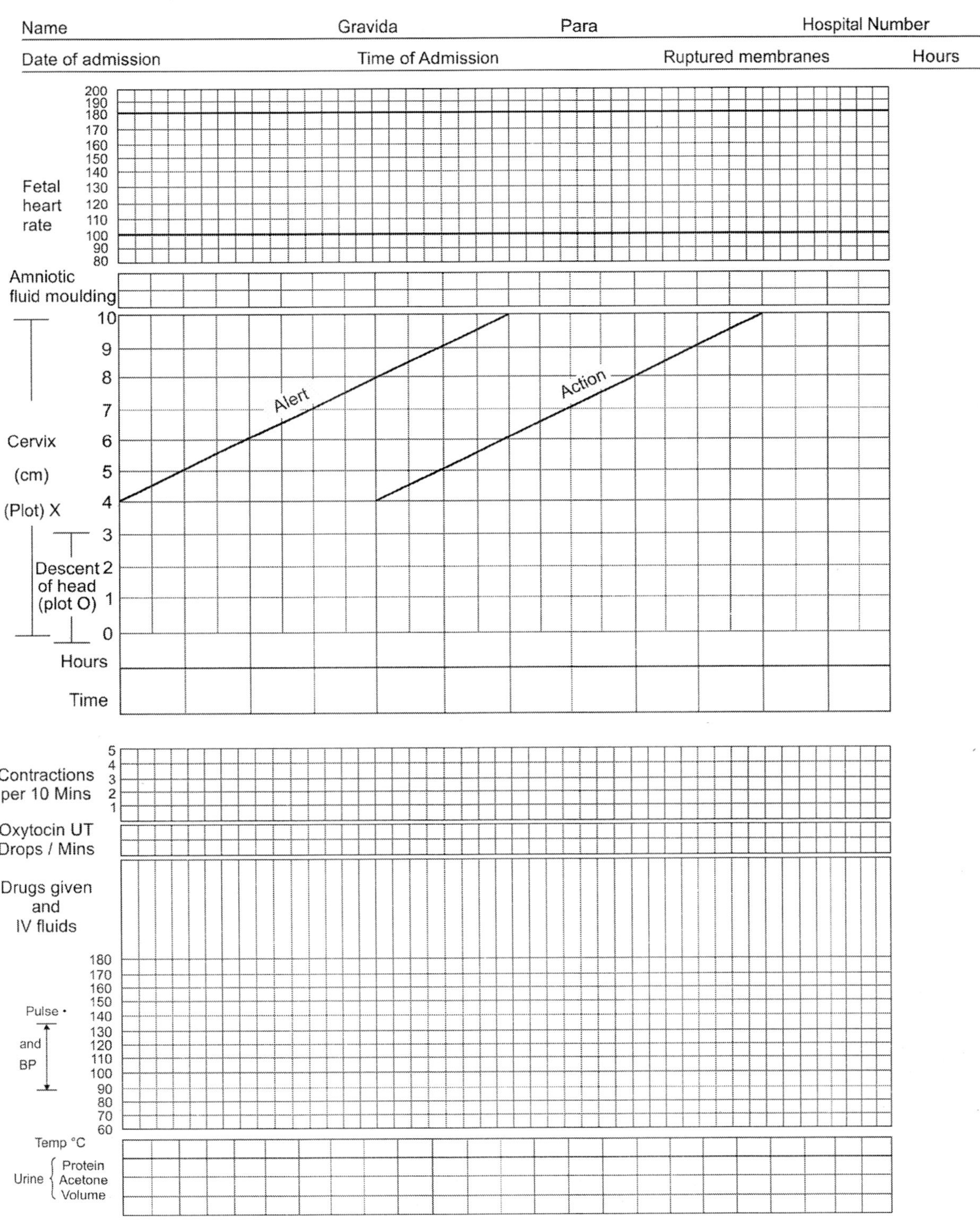
Name
Gravida
Para
Hospital Number
Date of admission
Time of Admission
Ruptured membranes
Hours
Fetal heart rate
200
190
180
170
160
150
140
130
120
110
100
90
80
Amniotic fluid moulding
Cervix (cm) (Plot) X
10
9
8
7
6
5
4
3
2
1
0
Alert
Action
Descent of head (plot O)
Hours
Time
Contractions per 10 Mins
5
4
3
2
1
Oxytocin UT Drops / Mins
Drugs given and IV fluids
Pulse •
and BP
180
170
160
150
140
130
120
110
100
90
80
70
60
Temp °C
Urine
Protein
Acetone
Volume

LABOUR SUMMARY

Type of labour: Spont/Induced

Mode of delivery: Vaginal/Instrument

Length of Labour:

1st stage .... Hrs .... Mins

2nd stage .... Hrs .... Mins

3rd stage .... Hrs .... Mins

Delivered by:..

CONDUCTED CARE STUDY

IDENTIFICATION DATA

Name of the Mother:..

Reg.No:..

Age:..

Gravida:..

Parity:..

Date of Admission and Time:..

Date of Delivery and Time:..

Date of Discharge:..

PAST MENSTRUAL HISTORY

LMP ....EDD ....Cycle...

HEALTH HISTORY

1. Past Obstetrical History..

....

....

2. Present Pregnancy History
   - I-trimester..

     ....

     ....
   - II-trimester..

     ....

     ....
   - III-trimester..

     ....

     ....

3. Past Medical History ....

....

....

4. Present Surgical History. ....

....

....

5. Past Surgical History. ....

....

....

6. Family History. ....

....

....

7. Personal History. ....

....

....

OBSTETRICAL HISTORY

S.No.	Year	Abortion	Prem	F.T.	Type of Labour and Mode of Delivery	Gender	Live or Still Birth	Remark

INVESTIGATION

USG Date: ....Finding: BPD..

FL/CRL...

Blood Group: .... Hb: .... Urine: ALB...................... Placenta...

RH Factor: .... VDRL:..................................... Sug.................... .... Gest. Wks..

Liquor...

Anamoly...

ANTENATAL ATTENDANCES							
LMP............................ EDD...Gestation at 1st visit.................. wk							
Date	Wt	BP	FHS	Weeks	Fundal height	Presentation	Treatments and Remarks

Labour Ward Admission Notes:

Admitted on:...at .... AM/PM

Contraction Commenced on: ....at .... AM/PM

Period of Gestation:...weeks

Height of Fundus..cms.

Presentation:..

Position: ....

Engaged /Not Engaged:

FHS:... /min

Bladder: Voided/Catheter

Bowel: SE Given/Not Given (Reason)

Remarks if Any:..

LABOUR RECORD : 1st STAGE

I.	**OBSERVATION**										
	UTERINE CONTRATION										
	a. Frequency in 10 mins										
	b. Duration in Secs										
	c. Intensity										
II.	**PER VAGINAL EXAM**										
	a. Cervical Dilatation										
	b. Cer. Effacement										
	c. Membranes										
	d. Presentation Part										
	e. Station										
	f. Position of Occiput										
	PARAMETERS										
	be. FHS/min										
III.	bf. Pulse/min										
	bg. BP										
	bh. Urine output										
IV.	**MEDICATION**										
V.	**SUPPORTIVE TREATMENT**										

IInd Stage

Membranes Ruptured at..AM/PM Spont/Artificial

Colour of Liqour..

Full Dilation /Explusive Cont Began at ....AM/PM On..

MOTHER:

Perineum: Rigid/Lax

Episiotomy: Given /Not Given

NEONATE:

Born at: ....AM/PM

On:...

Gender: Male/Female

Apgar Score 1min: ....

5 min: ....

Complication:

Treatment: Airway: ....

Eyes:..

Cord: ....

IIIrd Stage

a. Placenta and Membranes:

Delivered at.. AM/PM

Complete/Incomplete

Cord Insertion: Central/Marginal/Velamentous

Cord Length: .... (Inches)

Weight:...

b. Condition of Uterus:

c. PERINEUM: Episiotomy/Tear Laceration

Repair:..No.of Sutures ....No.of Catgut

d. Drugs given: ....

e. Approximate blood loss ....ml

PARTOGRAPH

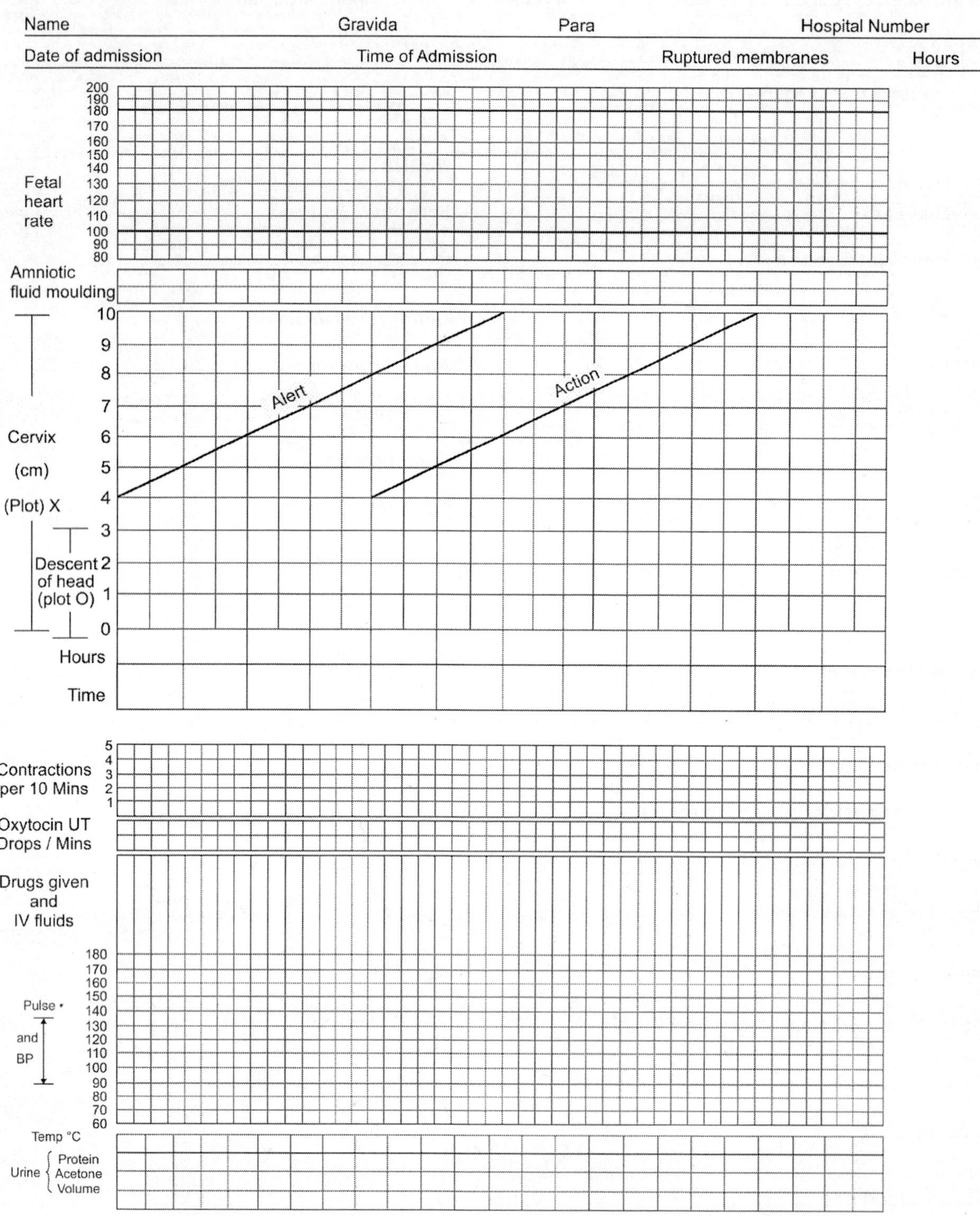
Name
Gravida
Para
Hospital Number
Date of admission
Time of Admission
Ruptured membranes
Hours
Fetal heart rate
200
190
180
170
160
150
140
130
120
110
100
90
80
Amniotic fluid moulding
Cervix (cm) (Plot) X
10
9
8
7
6
5
4
3
2
1
0
Alert
Action
Descent of head (plot O)
Hours
Time
Contractions per 10 Mins
5
4
3
2
1
Oxytocin UT Drops / Mins
Drugs given and IV fluids
Pulse •
and BP
180
170
160
150
140
130
120
110
100
90
80
70
60
Temp °C
Urine
Protein
Acetone
Volume

LABOUR SUMMARY

Type of labour: Spont/Induced

Mode of delivery: Vaginal/Instrument

Length of Labour:

1st stage .... Hrs .... Mins

2nd stage .... Hrs .... Mins

3rd stage .... Hrs .... Mins

Delivered by: ....

CONDUCTED CARE STUDY

IDENTIFICATION DATA

Name of the Mother:..

Reg.No:..

Age:..

Gravida:..

Parity:..

Date of Admission and Time:..

Date of Delivery and Time:..

Date of Discharge:..

PAST MENSTRUAL HISTORY

LMP .... EDD .... Cycle ....

HEALTH HISTORY

1. Past Obstetrical History..

....

....

2. Present Pregnancy History

- I-trimester..

....

....

- II-trimester..

....

....

- III-trimester..

....

....

3. Past Medical History ....

....

....

4. Present Surgical History. ....

....

....

5. Past Surgical History. ....

....

....

6. Family History. ....

....

....

7. Personal History. ....

....

....

OBSTETRICAL HISTORY

S.No.	Year	Abortion	Prem	F.T.	Type of Labour and Mode of Delivery	Gender	Live or Still Birth	Remark

INVESTIGATION

USG Date: ....Finding: BPD..

FL/CRL..

Blood Group: .... Hb: .... Urine: ALB .... Placenta ....

RH Factor: .... VDRL:.................................... Sug.................. .... Gest. Wks ....

Liquor ....

Anamoly ....

ANTENATAL ATTENDANCES

LMP............................ EDD...Gestation at 1st visit.................. wk

Date	Wt	BP	FHS	Weeks	Fundal height	Presentation	Treatments and Remarks

Labour Ward Admission Notes:

Admitted on:..at .... AM/PM

Contraction Commenced on: ....at .... AM/PM

Period of Gestation:...weeks

Height of Fundus ....cms.

Presentation:...

Position: ....

Engaged /Not Engaged:

FHS:.. /min

Bladder: Voided/Catheter

Bowel: SE Given/Not Given (Reason)

Remarks if Any:..

LABOUR RECORD : 1st STAGE

I.	**OBSERVATION**										
	UTERINE CONTRATION										
	a. Frequency in 10 mins										
	b. Duration in Secs										
	c. Intensity										
II.	**PER VAGINAL EXAM**										
	a. Cervical Dilatation										
	b. Cer. Effacement										
	c. Membranes										
	d. Presentation Part										
	e. Station										
	f. Position of Occiput										
III.	**PARAMETERS**										
	bi. FHS/min										
	bj. Pulse/min										
	bk. BP										
	bl. Urine output										
IV.	**MEDICATION**										
V.	**SUPPORTIVE TREATMENT**										

IInd Stage

Membranes Ruptured at...AM/PM Spont/Artificial

Colour of Liqour..

Full Dilation /Explusive Cont Began at ....AM/PM On...

MOTHER:

Perineum: Rigid/Lax

Episiotomy: Given /Not Given

NEONATE:

Born at: ....AM/PM

On:..

Gender: Male/Female

Apgar Score 1min:..

5 min: ....

Complication:

Treatment: Airway:.......................................

Eyes:..

Cord:...

IIIrd Stage

a. Placenta and Membranes:

Delivered at.. AM/PM

Complete/Incomplete

Cord Insertion: Central/Marginal/Velamentous

Cord Length: .... (Inches)

Weight:..

b. Condition of Uterus:

c. PERINEUM: Episiotomy/Tear Laceration

Repair:...No.of Sutures ....No.of Catgut

d. Drugs given: ....

e. Approximate blood loss ....ml

PARTOGRAPH

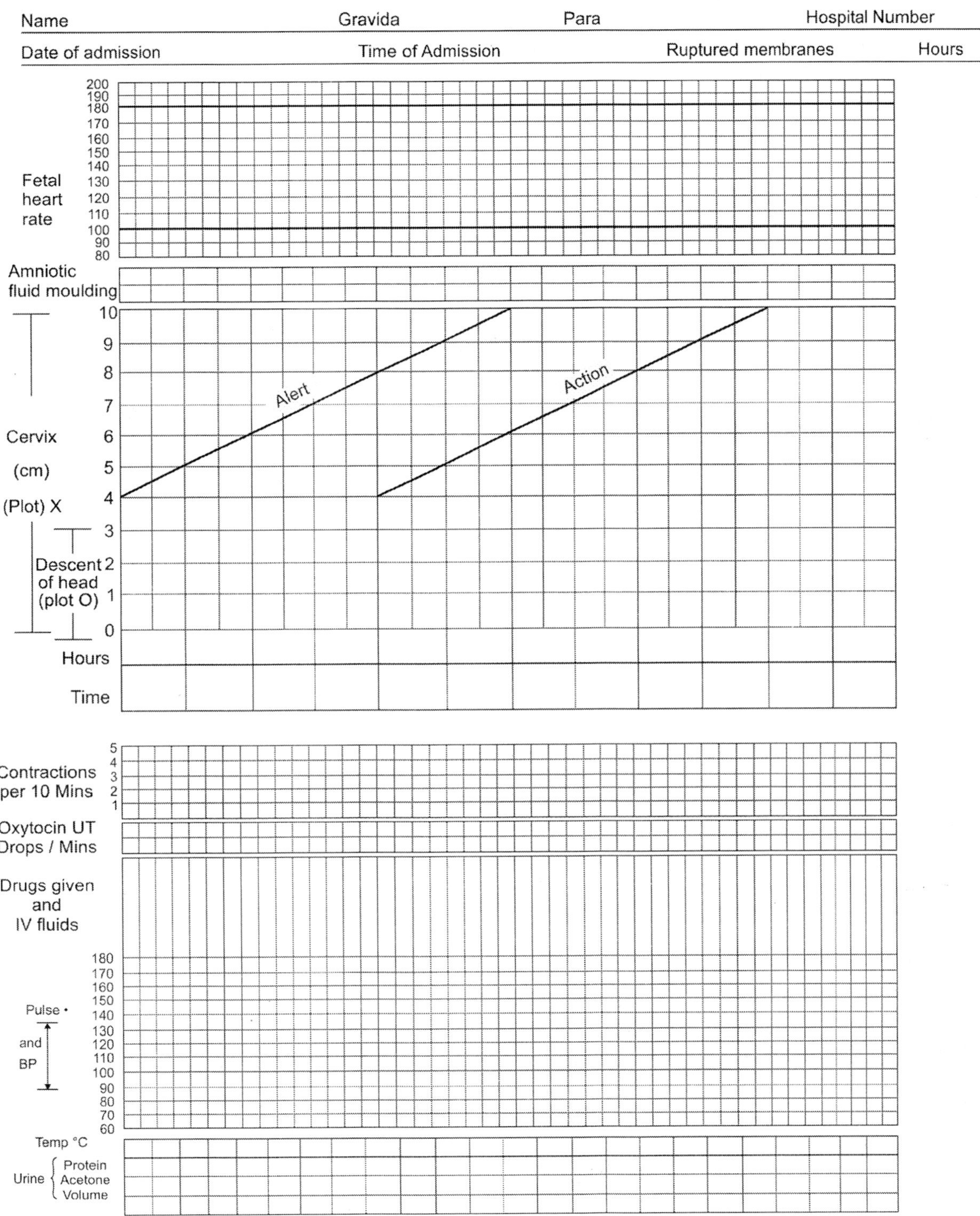
Name
Gravida
Para
Hospital Number
Date of admission
Time of Admission
Ruptured membranes
Hours
Fetal heart rate
200
190
180
170
160
150
140
130
120
110
100
90
80
Amniotic fluid moulding
Cervix (cm) (Plot) X
10
9
8
7
6
5
4
3
2
1
0
Alert
Action
Descent of head (plot O)
Hours
Time
Contractions per 10 Mins
5
4
3
2
1
Oxytocin UT Drops / Mins
Drugs given and IV fluids
Pulse •
and
BP
180
170
160
150
140
130
120
110
100
90
80
70
60
Temp °C
Urine
Protein
Acetone
Volume

LABOUR SUMMARY

Type of labour: Spont/Induced

Mode of delivery: Vaginal/Instrument

Length of Labour:

1st stage .... Hrs .... Mins

2nd stage .... Hrs .... Mins

3rd stage .... Hrs .... Mins

Delivered by: ....

CONDUCTED CARE STUDY

IDENTIFICATION DATA

Name of the Mother:...

Reg.No:...

Age:...

Gravida:...

Parity:...

Date of Admission and Time:...

Date of Delivery and Time:...

Date of Discharge:...

PAST MENSTRUAL HISTORY

LMP .... EDD .... Cycle..

HEALTH HISTORY

1. Past Obstetrical History...

   ....

   ....

2. Present Pregnancy History

   - I-trimester...

     ....

     ....

   - II-trimester...

     ....

     ....

   - III-trimester...

     ....

     ....

3. Past Medical History ....

....

....

4. Present Surgical History. ....

....

....

5. Past Surgical History. ....

....

....

6. Family History. ....

....

....

7. Personal History. ....

....

....

OBSTETRICAL HISTORY

S.No.	Year	Abortion	Prem	F.T.	Type of Labour and Mode of Delivery	Gender	Live or Still Birth	Remark

INVESTIGATION

USG Date: ....Finding: BPD..

FL/CRL..

Blood Group: .... Hb: .... Urine: ALB...................... Placenta...

RH Factor: .... VDRL:..................................... Sug.................. ....Gest. Wks..

Liquor...

Anamoly..

ANTENATAL ATTENDANCES

LMP............................ EDD..Gestation at 1st visit.................. wk

Date	Wt	BP	FHS	Weeks	Fundal height	Presentation	Treatments and Remarks

Labour Ward Admission Notes:

Admitted on:...at .... AM/PM

Contraction Commenced on: ....at .... AM/PM

Period of Gestation:...weeks

Height of Fundus..cms.

Presentation:...

Position: ....

Engaged /Not Engaged:

FHS:.. /min

Bladder: Voided/Catheter

Bowel: SE Given/Not Given (Reason)

Remarks if Any:..

LABOUR RECORD : 1st STAGE

I.	**OBSERVATION**										
	UTERINE CONTRATION										
	a. Frequency in 10 mins										
	b. Duration in Secs										
	c. Intensity										
II.	**PER VAGINAL EXAM**										
	a. Cervical Dilatation										
	b. Cer. Effacement										
	c. Membranes										
	d. Presentation Part										
	e. Station										
	f. Position of Occiput										
	PARAMETERS										
	bm. FHS/min										
III.	bn. Pulse/min										
	bo. BP										
	bp. Urine output										
IV.	**MEDICATION**										
V.	**SUPPORTIVE TREATMENT**										

IInd Stage

Membranes Ruptured at..AM/PM Spont/Artificial

Colour of Liqour..

Full Dilation /Explusive Cont Began at ....AM/PM On...

MOTHER:

Perineum: Rigid/Lax

Episiotomy: Given /Not Given

NEONATE:

Born at: ....AM/PM

On: ....

Gender: Male/Female

Apgar Score 1min: ....

5 min: ....

Complication:

Treatment: Airway: ....

Eyes: ....

Cord: ....

IIIrd Stage

a. Placenta and Membranes:

Delivered at .... AM/PM

Complete/Incomplete

Cord Insertion: Central/Marginal/Velamentous

Cord Length: .... (Inches)

Weight: ....

b. Condition of Uterus:

c. PERINEUM: Episiotomy/Tear Laceration

Repair: ....No.of Sutures ....No.of Catgut

d. Drugs given: ....

e. Approximate blood loss ....ml

PARTOGRAPH

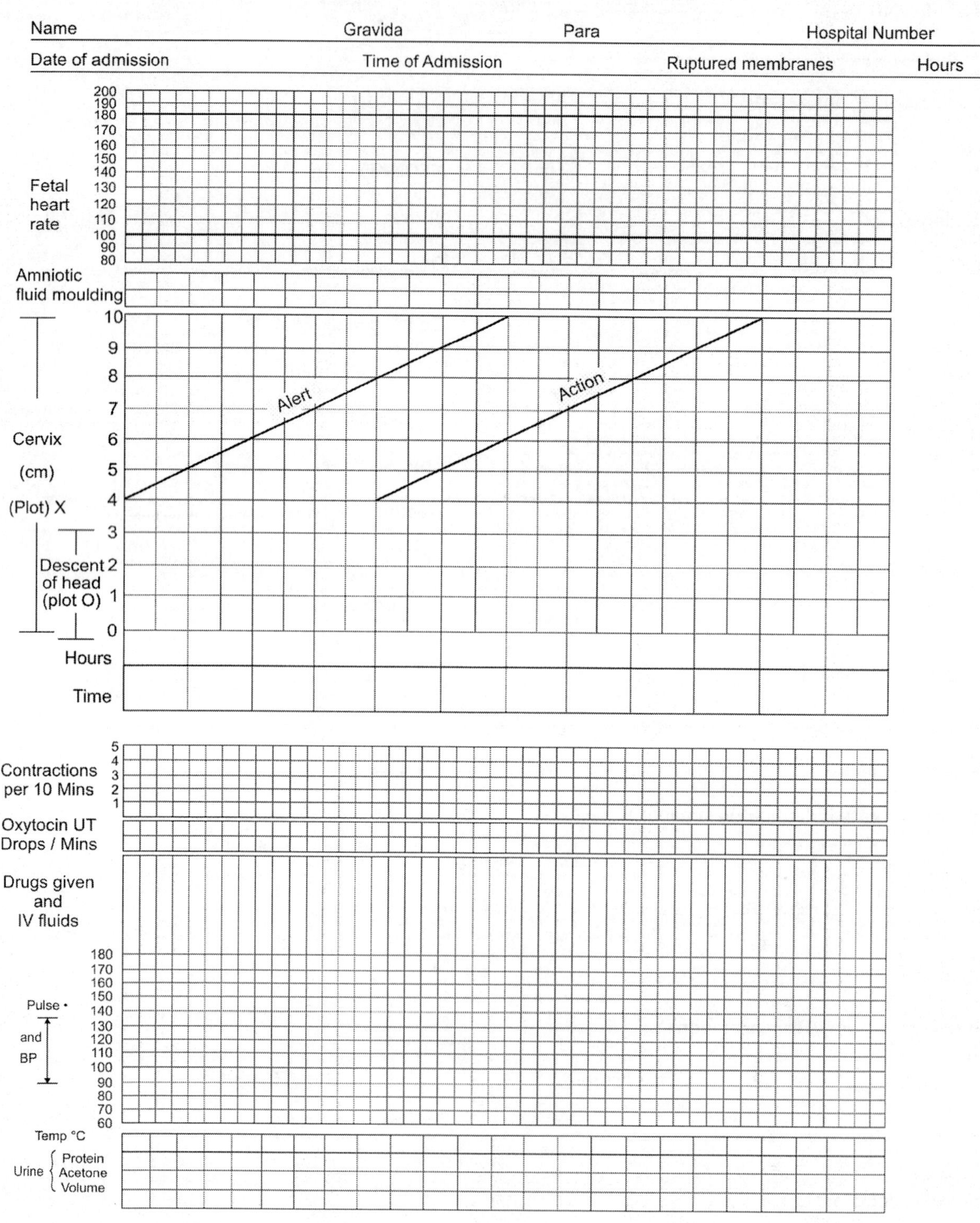
Name
Gravida
Para
Hospital Number
Date of admission
Time of Admission
Ruptured membranes
Hours
200
190
180
170
160
150
140
130
120
110
100
90
80
Fetal heart rate
Amniotic fluid moulding
10
9
8
7
6
5
4
3
2
1
0
Alert
Action
Cervix (cm) (Plot) X
Descent of head (plot O)
Hours
Time
5
4
3
2
1
Contractions per 10 Mins
Oxytocin UT Drops / Mins
Drugs given and IV fluids
180
170
160
150
140
130
120
110
100
90
80
70
60
Pulse •
and BP
Temp °C
Urine
Protein
Acetone
Volume

LABOUR SUMMARY

Type of labour: Spont/Induced

Mode of delivery: Vaginal/Instrument

Length of Labour:

1st stage .... Hrs .... Mins

2nd stage .... Hrs .... Mins

3rd stage .... Hrs .... Mins

Delivered by: ....

CONDUCTED CARE STUDY

IDENTIFICATION DATA

Name of the Mother:...

Reg.No:..

Age:...

Gravida:...

Parity:..

Date of Admission and Time: ....

Date of Delivery and Time:..

Date of Discharge:..

PAST MENSTRUAL HISTORY

LMP ....EDD ....Cycle..

HEALTH HISTORY

1. Past Obstetrical History...

   ....

   ....

2. Present Pregnancy History

   - I-trimester ....

     ....

     ....

   - II-trimester ....

     ....

     ....

   - III-trimester ....

     ....

     ....

3. Past Medical History ....

....

....

4. Present Surgical History. ....

....

....

5. Past Surgical History. ....

....

....

6. Family History. ....

....

....

7. Personal History. ....

....

....

OBSTETRICAL HISTORY

S.No.	Year	Abortion	Prem	F.T.	Type of Labour and Mode of Delivery	Gender	Live or Still Birth	Remark

INVESTIGATION

USG Date: .... Finding: BPD..

FL/CRL..

Blood Group: .... Hb: .... Urine: ALB .... Placenta...

RH Factor: .... VDRL:.................................... Sug.................. .... Gest. Wks..

Liquor...

Anamoly..

ANTENATAL ATTENDANCES

LMP.............................. EDD...Gestation at 1st visit.................. wk

Date	Wt	BP	FHS	Weeks	Fundal height	Presentation	Treatments and Remarks

Labour Ward Admission Notes:

Admitted on:.. at .... AM/PM

Contraction Commenced on: .... at .... AM/PM

Period of Gestation:.. weeks

Height of Fundus.. cms.

Presentation:...

Position: ....

Engaged /Not Engaged:

FHS:.. /min

Bladder: Voided/Catheter

Bowel: SE Given/Not Given (Reason)

Remarks if Any:...

LABOUR RECORD : 1st STAGE

I.	**OBSERVATION**										
	UTERINE CONTRATION										
	a. Frequency in 10 mins										
	b. Duration in Secs										
	c. Intensity										
II.	**PER VAGINAL EXAM**										
	a. Cervical Dilatation										
	b. Cer. Effacement										
	c. Membranes										
	d. Presentation Part										
	e. Station										
	f. Position of Occiput										
III.	**PARAMETERS**										
	bq. FHS/min										
	br. Pulse/min										
	bs. BP										
	bt. Urine output										
IV.	**MEDICATION**										
V.	**SUPPORTIVE TREATMENT**										

IInd Stage

Membranes Ruptured at..AM/PM Spont/Artificial

Colour of Liqour..

Full Dilation /Explusive Cont Began at ....AM/PM On...

MOTHER:

Perineum: Rigid/Lax

Episiotomy: Given /Not Given

NEONATE:

Born at: ....AM/PM

On:..

Gender: Male/Female

Apgar Score 1min:..

5 min: ....

Complication:

Treatment: Airway:..

Eyes:...

Cord:...

IIIrd Stage

a. Placenta and Membranes:

Delivered at.. AM/PM

Complete/Incomplete

Cord Insertion: Central/Marginal/Velamentous

Cord Length: .... (Inches)

Weight:..

b. Condition of Uterus:

c. PERINEUM: Episiotomy/Tear Laceration

Repair:...No.of Sutures ....No.of Catgut

d. Drugs given: ....

e. Approximate blood loss ....ml

PARTOGRAPH

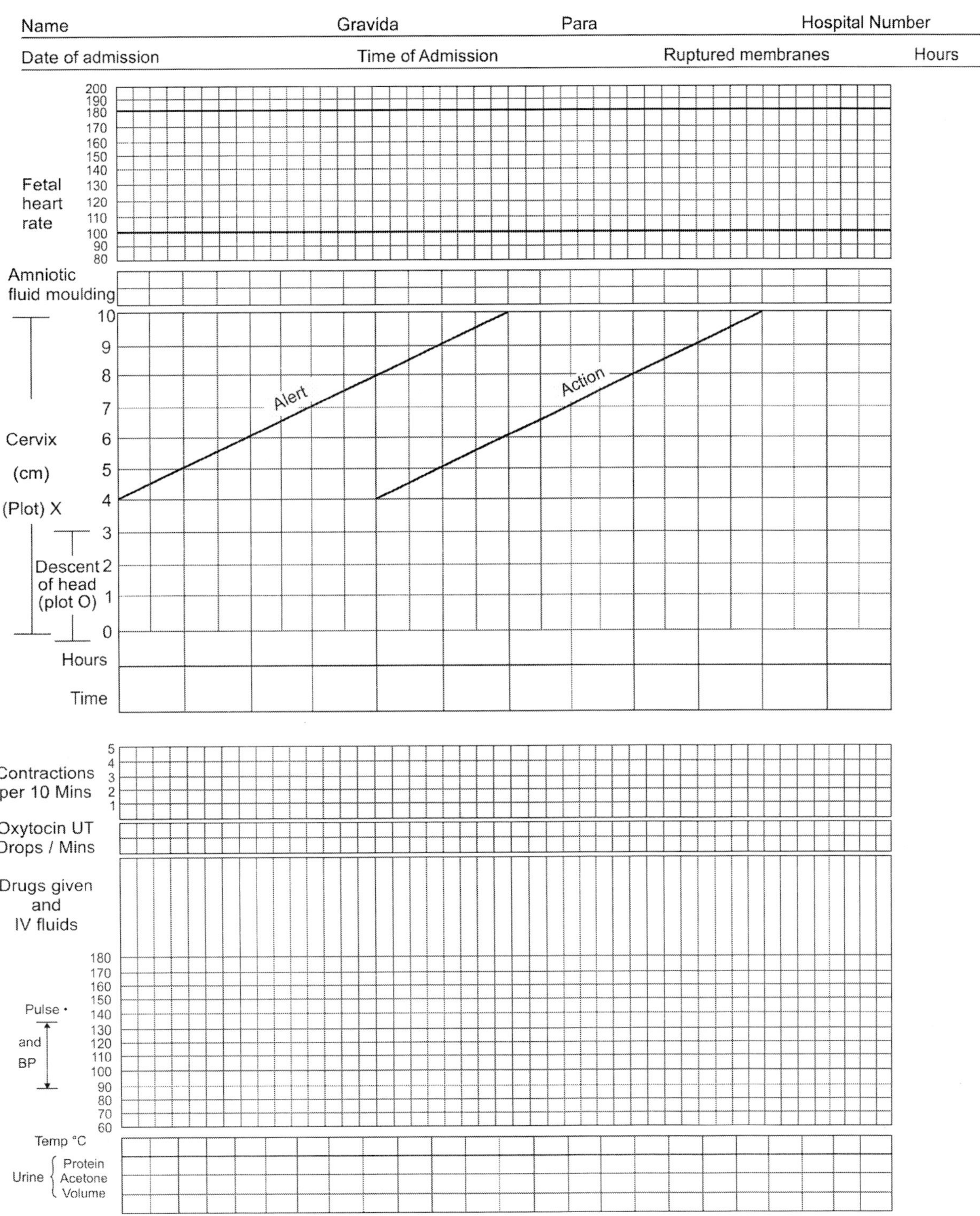
Name
Gravida
Para
Hospital Number
Date of admission
Time of Admission
Ruptured membranes
Hours
Fetal heart rate
200
190
180
170
160
150
140
130
120
110
100
90
80
Amniotic fluid moulding
10
9
8
7
6
5
4
3
2
1
0
Alert
Action
Cervix (cm) (Plot) X
Descent of head (plot O)
Hours
Time
Contractions per 10 Mins
5
4
3
2
1
Oxytocin UT Drops / Mins
Drugs given and IV fluids
Pulse •
and BP
180
170
160
150
140
130
120
110
100
90
80
70
60
Temp °C
Urine
Protein
Acetone
Volume

LABOUR SUMMARY

Type of labour: Spont/Induced

Mode of delivery: Vaginal/Instrument

Length of Labour:

1st stage .... Hrs .... Mins

2nd stage .... Hrs .... Mins

3rd stage .... Hrs .... Mins

Delivered by: ....

CONDUCTED CARE STUDY

IDENTIFICATION DATA

Name of the Mother:..

Reg.No:..

Age:..

Gravida:..

Parity:..

Date of Admission and Time:..

Date of Delivery and Time:..

Date of Discharge:..

PAST MENSTRUAL HISTORY

LMP ....EDD ....Cycle...

HEALTH HISTORY

1. Past Obstetrical History..

....

....

2. Present Pregnancy History

    - I-trimester..

      ....

      ....

    - II-trimester..

      ....

      ....

    - III-trimester..

      ....

      ....

3. Past Medical History ....

....

....

4. Present Surgical History. ....

....

....

5. Past Surgical History. ....

....

....

6. Family History. ....

....

....

7. Personal History. ....

....

....

OBSTETRICAL HISTORY

S.No.	Year	Abortion	Prem	F.T.	Type of Labour and Mode of Delivery	Gender	Live or Still Birth	Remark

INVESTIGATION

USG Date: ....Finding: BPD...

FL/CRL..

Blood Group: .... Hb: .... Urine: ALB...................... Placenta...

RH Factor: .... VDRL:.................................... Sug.................. ....Gest. Wks...

Liquor...

Anamoly...

ANTENATAL ATTENDANCES							
LMP............................. EDD..Gestation at 1st visit.................. wk							
Date	Wt	BP	FHS	Weeks	Fundal height	Presentation	Treatments and Remarks

Labour Ward Admission Notes:

Admitted on:..at .... AM/PM

Contraction Commenced on: ....at .... AM/PM

Period of Gestation:...weeks

Height of Fundus ....cms.

Presentation:...

Position: ....

Engaged /Not Engaged:

FHS:.. /min

Bladder: Voided/Catheter

Bowel: SE Given/Not Given (Reason)

Remarks if Any:..

LABOUR RECORD : 1st STAGE

I.	**OBSERVATION**										
	UTERINE CONTRATION										
	a. Frequency in 10 mins										
	b. Duration in Secs										
	c. Intensity										
II.	**PER VAGINAL EXAM**										
	a. Cervical Dilatation										
	b. Cer. Effacement										
	c. Membranes										
	d. Presentation Part										
	e. Station										
	f. Position of Occiput										
	PARAMETERS										
	bu. FHS/min										
III.	bv. Pulse/min										
	bw. BP										
	bx. Urine output										
IV.	**MEDICATION**										
V.	**SUPPORTIVE TREATMENT**										

IInd Stage

Membranes Ruptured at..AM/PM Spont/Artificial

Colour of Liqour..

Full Dilation /Explusive Cont Began at ....AM/PM On...

MOTHER:

Perineum: Rigid/Lax

Episiotomy: Given /Not Given

NEONATE:

Born at: ....AM/PM

On:...

Gender: Male/Female

Apgar Score 1min: ....

5 min: ....

Complication:

Treatment: Airway: ....

Eyes:...

Cord: ....

IIIrd Stage

a. Placenta and Membranes:

Delivered at .... AM/PM

Complete/Incomplete

Cord Insertion: Central/Marginal/Velamentous

Cord Length: .... (Inches)

Weight:...

b. Condition of Uterus:

c. PERINEUM: Episiotomy/Tear Laceration

Repair:..No.of Sutures ....No.of Catgut

d. Drugs given: ....

e. Approximate blood loss ....ml

PARTOGRAPH

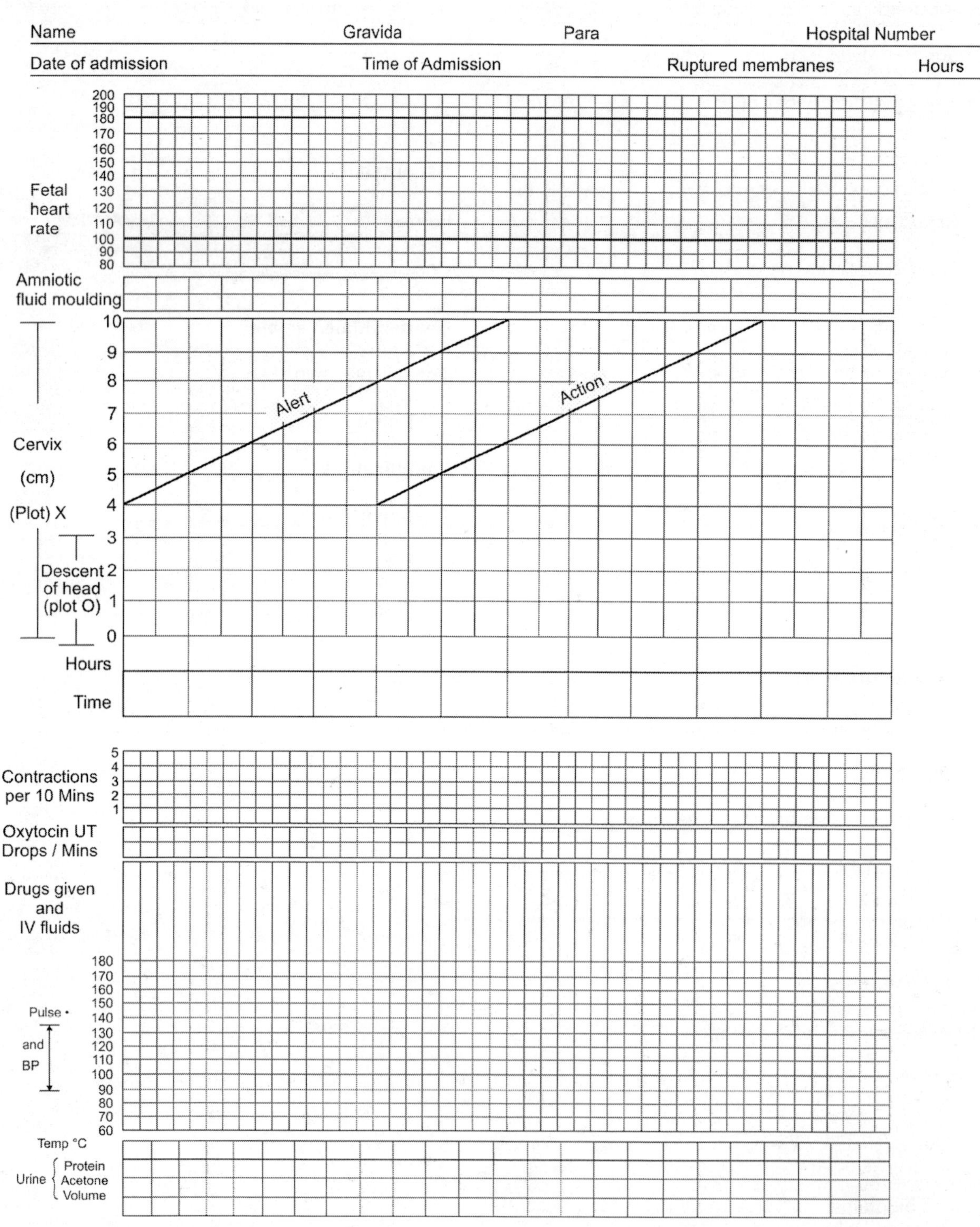
Name
Gravida
Para
Hospital Number
Date of admission
Time of Admission
Ruptured membranes
Hours
Fetal heart rate
200
190
180
170
160
150
140
130
120
110
100
90
80
Amniotic fluid moulding
Cervix (cm) (Plot) X
10
9
8
7
6
5
4
3
2
1
0
Alert
Action
Descent of head (plot O)
Hours
Time
Contractions per 10 Mins
5
4
3
2
1
Oxytocin UT Drops / Mins
Drugs given and IV fluids
Pulse •
and BP
180
170
160
150
140
130
120
110
100
90
80
70
60
Temp °C
Urine
Protein
Acetone
Volume

LABOUR SUMMARY

Type of labour: Spont/Induced

Mode of delivery: Vaginal/Instrument

Length of Labour:

1st stage .... Hrs .... Mins

2nd stage .... Hrs .... Mins

3rd stage .... Hrs .... Mins

Delivered by: ....

CONDUCTED CARE STUDY

IDENTIFICATION DATA

Name of the Mother:..

Reg.No: ....

Age:..

Gravida: ....

Parity: ....

Date of Admission and Time: ....

Date of Delivery and Time:..

Date of Discharge:..

PAST MENSTRUAL HISTORY

LMP ....EDD ....Cycle..

HEALTH HISTORY

1. Past Obstetrical History..

   ....

   ....

2. Present Pregnancy History

   - I-trimester ....

     ....

     ....

   - II-trimester ....

     ....

     ....

   - III-trimester..

     ....

     ....

3. Past Medical History ....

....

....

4. Present Surgical History. ....

....

....

5. Past Surgical History. ....

....

....

6. Family History. ....

....

....

7. Personal History. ....

....

....

OBSTETRICAL HISTORY

S.No.	Year	Abortion	Prem	F.T.	Type of Labour and Mode of Delivery	Gender	Live or Still Birth	Remark

INVESTIGATION

USG Date: ....Finding: BPD..

FL/CRL..

Blood Group: .... Hb: .... Urine: ALB .... Placenta ....

RH Factor: .... VDRL:................................... Sug.................. .... Gest. Wks ....

Liquor ....

Anamoly ....

ANTENATAL ATTENDANCES

LMP............................ EDD...Gestation at 1st visit.................. wk

Date	Wt	BP	FHS	Weeks	Fundal height	Presentation	Treatments and Remarks

Labour Ward Admission Notes:

Admitted on:.. at .... AM/PM

Contraction Commenced on: .... at .... AM/PM

Period of Gestation:..weeks

Height of Fundus ....cms.

Presentation:..

Position: ....

Engaged /Not Engaged:

FHS:.. /min

Bladder: Voided/Catheter

Bowel: SE Given/Not Given (Reason)

Remarks if Any:..

LABOUR RECORD : 1st STAGE

I.	**OBSERVATION**										
	UTERINE CONTRATION										
	a. Frequency in 10 mins										
	b. Duration in Secs										
	c. Intensity										
II.	**PER VAGINAL EXAM**										
	a. Cervical Dilatation										
	b. Cer. Effacement										
	c. Membranes										
	d. Presentation Part										
	e. Station										
	f. Position of Occiput										
	PARAMETERS										
	by. FHS/min										
III.	bz. Pulse/min										
	ca. BP										
	cb. Urine output										
IV.	**MEDICATION**										
V.	**SUPPORTIVE TREATMENT**										

IInd Stage

Membranes Ruptured at...AM/PM Spont/Artificial

Colour of Liqour..

Full Dilation /Explusive Cont Began at ....AM/PM On..

MOTHER:

Perineum: Rigid/Lax

Episiotomy: Given /Not Given

NEONATE:

Born at: ....AM/PM

On:...

Gender: Male/Female

Apgar Score 1min:..

5 min: ....

Complication:

Treatment: Airway:.......................................

Eyes:...

Cord:...

IIIrd Stage

a. Placenta and Membranes:

Delivered at.. AM/PM

Complete/Incomplete

Cord Insertion: Central/Marginal/Velamentous

Cord Length: .... (Inches)

Weight:..

b. Condition of Uterus:

c. PERINEUM: Episiotomy/Tear Laceration

Repair:..No.of Sutures ....No.of Catgut

d. Drugs given: ....

e. Approximate blood loss ....ml

PARTOGRAPH

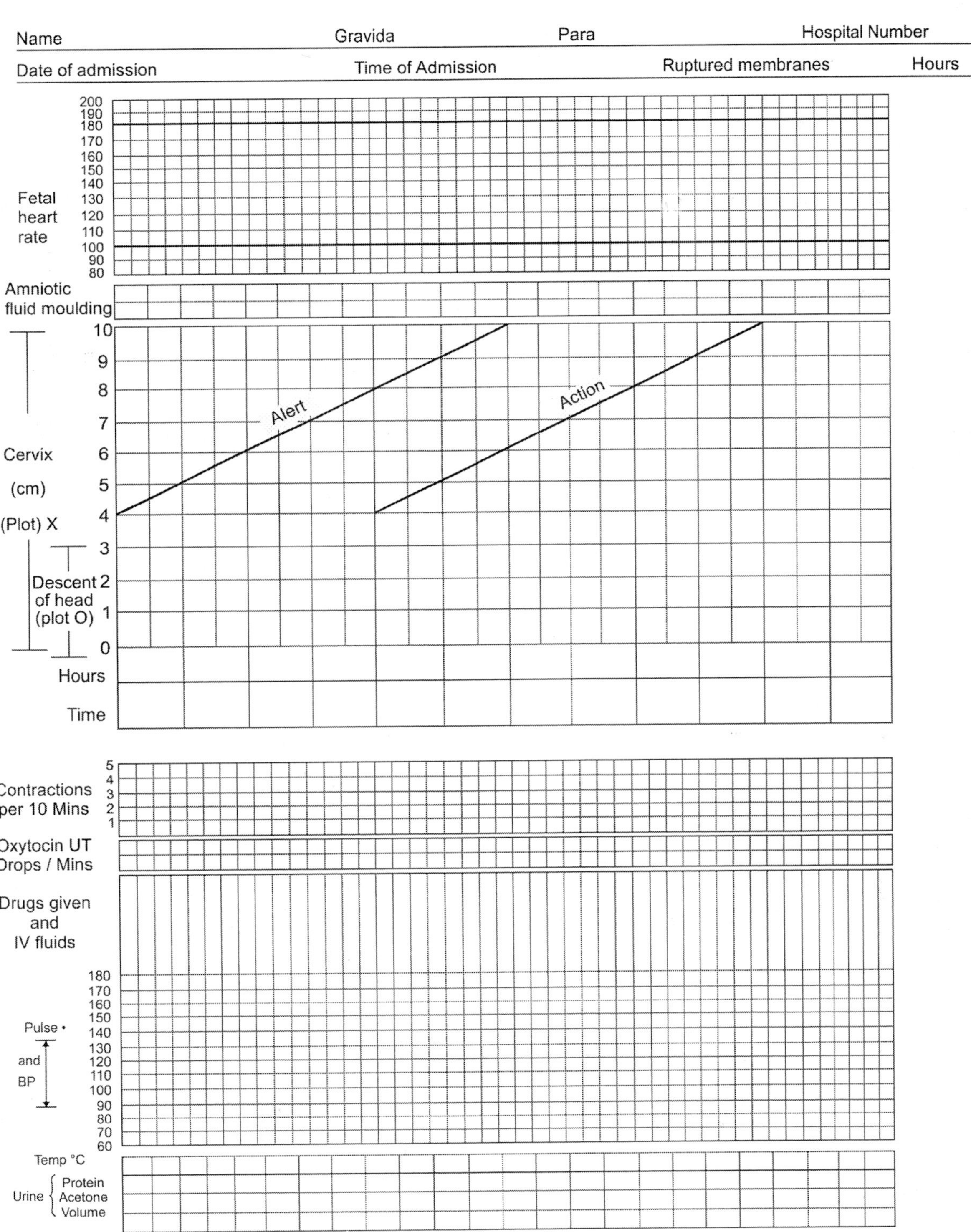
Name
Gravida
Para
Hospital Number
Date of admission
Time of Admission
Ruptured membranes
Hours
Fetal heart rate
200
190
180
170
160
150
140
130
120
110
100
90
80
Amniotic fluid moulding
Cervix (cm) (Plot) X
10
9
8
7
6
5
4
3
2
1
0
Alert
Action
Descent of head (plot O)
Hours
Time
Contractions per 10 Mins
5
4
3
2
1
Oxytocin UT Drops / Mins
Drugs given and IV fluids
Pulse •
and BP
180
170
160
150
140
130
120
110
100
90
80
70
60
Temp °C
Urine
Protein
Acetone
Volume

LABOUR SUMMARY

Type of labour: Spont/Induced

Mode of delivery: Vaginal/Instrument

Length of Labour:

1st stage .... Hrs .... Mins

2nd stage .... Hrs .... Mins

3rd stage .... Hrs .... Mins

Delivered by: ....

POSTNATAL AND NEONATAL CARE STUDY

IDENTIFICATION DATA

Name of Mother:..
W/o: ....
Age:..
Ward Name/Bed Number:...
Address: ....
Date of Admission:...
Date of Discharge:..
Obstetrical History – GPLA: ....

PAST MENSTRUAL HISTORY

LMP ....EDD ....Cycle..

HEALTH HISTORY

1. Past Obstetrical History...
....
....
2. Present Pregnancy History
   - I-trimester ....
   ....
   ....
   - II-trimester ....
   ....
   ....
   - III-trimester..
   ....
   ....
3. Past Medical History ....
....
....
4. Present Surgical History. ....
....
....
5. Past Surgical History. ....
....
....

6. Family History. ....
....
....

7. Personal History. ....
....
....

OBSTETRICAL HISTORY

S.No.	Year	Abortion	Prem	FT	Type of labour and mode of delivery	Gender	Live or Still Birth	Remark

LAB -INVESTIGATION

Hb	Blood Grouping	Blood Sugar	Urine		HIV	VDRL	Any Other
			Albumin	Sugar			

THE PUERPERIUM

Admitted to Postnatal Ward at AM/PM On:

POSTNATAL OBSERVATION CHART FOR MOTHER

Date	Day	Weight	Temp	Pulse	Resp	Fundal Height	Bowel	Urine	Lochia	Breast	Episiotomy Wound	Homen-sign

DELIVERY/OPERATION NOTES

Normal Vaginal Delivery

Type of labour : Spont /induced ....

Mode of delivery: Normal ....

Instrumental ....

Forcep/Vaccum ....

Indication: ....

Operation notes ....

....

....

....

....

....

....

CAESAREAN SECTION

Elective /Emergency...

Indication ....

Type: Lower Segment/Classical ....

Anaesthesia: Ga/Spinal/Epidural ....

Surgical Note...

1st Stage:..............................Hrs..Mins.

2nd Stage:............................Hrs..Mins.

3rd Stage: ....Hrs..Mins.

Total : ....Hrs..Mins.

NEWBORN ASSESSMENT

Name of Baby.. Gender.................................. Age...........

Apgar Score .... 1min ....5 min Condition: Poor/Fair/Good

OBSERVATION CHART-BABY						
Date						
Day						
Weight						
Skin Colour						
Cord						
Eyes						
Mouth						
Urine						
Meconium						
Feeds						
Temperature						
Heart Rate						
Respiration						

Measurement:

Length ....cm

Head Circumference..cm

Chest Circumference..cm

Abdominal Circumference...cm

Reflexes:

Moro: ....

Sucking: ....

Swallowing: ....

Rooting:..

Grasping: ....

Vaccination: Age of the Baby...

BCG-Yes/No...

OPV-Yes/No...

Hep B-Yes/No ....

NURSING PROBLEMS AND RELATED OBJECTIVE OF CARE

Actual Nursing Problem for Mother and Baby

....

....

....

....

....

Potential Nursing Problems for Mother and Baby

....

....

....

....

NURSING CARE PLAN

ASSESSMENT	NSG DIAGNOSIS	GOAL	PLANNING	IMPLEMENTATION

Health Education to Mother

....

....

....

....

....

....

POSTNATAL AND NEONATAL CARE STUDY

IDENTIFICATION DATA

Name of Mother:..
W/o:..
Age:..
Ward Name/Bed Number:..
Address:..
Date of Admission:..
Date of Discharge:..
Obstetrical History – GPLA:..

PAST MENSTRUAL HISTORY

LMP ....EDD ....Cycle..

HEALTH HISTORY

1. Past Obstetrical History..
....
....
2. Present Pregnancy History
   - I-trimester..
   ....
   ....
   - II-trimester..
   ....
   ....
   - III-trimester..
   ....
   ....
3. Past Medical History..
....
....
4. Present Surgical History. ....
....
....
5. Past Surgical History. ....
....
....

6. Family History. ....
....
....

7. Personal History. ....
....
....

OBSTETRICAL HISTORY

S.No.	Year	Abortion	Prem	FT	Type of labour and mode of delivery	Gender	Live or Still Birth	Remark

LAB -INVESTIGATION

Hb	Blood Grouping	Blood Sugar	Urine		HIV	VDRL	Any Other
			Albumin	Sugar			

THE PUERPERIUM

Admitted to Postnatal Ward at AM/PM On:

POSTNATAL OBSERVATION CHART FOR MOTHER

Date	Day	Weight	Temp	Pulse	Resp	Fundal Height	Bowel	Urine	Lochia	Breast	Episiotomy Wound	Homen-sign

DELIVERY/OPERATION NOTES

Normal Vaginal Delivery

Type of labour : Spont /induced ....

Mode of delivery: Normal ....

Instrumental ....

Forcep/Vaccum ....

Indication: ....

Operation notes ....

....

....

....

....

....

....

CAESAREAN SECTION

Elective /Emergency..

Indication ....

Type: Lower Segment/Classical ....

Anaesthesia: Ga/Spinal/Epidural ....

Surgical Note..

1st Stage:..............................Hrs..Mins.

2nd Stage:............................Hrs..Mins.

3rd Stage: ....Hrs..Mins.

Total : ....Hrs..Mins.

NEWBORN ASSESSMENT

Name of Baby...Gender.................................. Age...........

Apgar Score .... 1min ....5 min Condition: Poor/Fair/Good

OBSERVATION CHART-BABY						
Date						
Day						
Weight						
Skin Colour						
Cord						
Eyes						
Mouth						
Urine						
Meconium						
Feeds						
Temperature						
Heart Rate						
Respiration						

Measurement:

Length ....cm

Head Circumference...cm

Chest Circumference..cm

Abdominal Circumference...cm

Reflexes:

Moro: ....

Sucking: ....

Swallowing: ....

Rooting:...

Grasping: ....

Vaccination: Age of the Baby..

BCG-Yes/No...

OPV-Yes/No...

Hep B-Yes/No ....

NURSING PROBLEMS AND RELATED OBJECTIVE OF CARE

Actual Nursing Problem for Mother and Baby

....

....

....

....

....

Potential Nursing Problems for Mother and Baby

....

....

....

....

NURSING CARE PLAN

ASSESSMENT	NSG DIAGNOSIS	GOAL	PLANNING	IMPLEMENTATION

Health Education to Mother

....

....

....

....

....

....

POSTNATAL AND NEONATAL CARE STUDY

IDENTIFICATION DATA

Name of Mother:..

W/o: ....

Age:..

Ward Name/Bed Number:..

Address: ....

Date of Admission:..

Date of Discharge:..

Obstetrical History – GPLA: ....

PAST MENSTRUAL HISTORY

LMP ....EDD ....Cycle...

HEALTH HISTORY

1. Past Obstetrical History..
   ....
   ....
2. Present Pregnancy History
   - I-trimester..
     ....
     ....
   - II-trimester..
     ....
     ....
   - III-trimester..
     ....
     ....
3. Past Medical History ....
   ....
   ....
4. Present Surgical History. ....
   ....
   ....
5. Past Surgical History. ....
   ....
   ....

6. Family History. ....
....
....

7. Personal History. ....
....
....

OBSTETRICAL HISTORY

S.No.	Year	Abortion	Prem	FT	Type of labour and mode of delivery	Gender	Live or Still Birth	Remark

LAB -INVESTIGATION

Hb	Blood Grouping	Blood Sugar	Urine		HIV	VDRL	Any Other
			Albumin	Sugar			

THE PUERPERIUM

Admitted to Postnatal Ward at AM/PM On:

POSTNATAL OBSERVATION CHART FOR MOTHER

Date	Day	Weight	Temp	Pulse	Resp	Fundal Height	Bowel	Urine	Lochia	Breast	Episiotomy Wound	Homen-sign

DELIVERY/OPERATION NOTES

Normal Vaginal Delivery

Type of labour : Spont /induced ....

Mode of delivery: Normal ....

Instrumental ....

Forcep/Vaccum..

Indication:..

Operation notes ....

....

....

....

....

....

....

CAESAREAN SECTION

Elective /Emergency..

Indication ....

Type: Lower Segment/Classical ....

Anaesthesia: Ga/Spinal/Epidural ....

Surgical Note...

1st Stage:..............................Hrs..Mins.

2nd Stage:............................Hrs..Mins.

3rd Stage:.............................Hrs..Mins.

Total : ....Hrs..Mins.

NEWBORN ASSESSMENT

Name of Baby... Gender................................... Age...........

Apgar Score .... 1min ....5 min Condition: Poor/Fair/Good

OBSERVATION CHART-BABY						
Date						
Day						
Weight						
Skin Colour						
Cord						
Eyes						
Mouth						
Urine						
Meconium						
Feeds						
Temperature						
Heart Rate						
Respiration						

Measurement:

Length ....cm

Head Circumference...cm

Chest Circumference..cm

Abdominal Circumference..cm

Reflexes:

Moro: ....

Sucking: ....

Swallowing: ....

Rooting:..

Grasping: ....

Vaccination: Age of the Baby..

BCG-Yes/No...

OPV-Yes/No...

Hep B-Yes/No ....

NURSING PROBLEMS AND RELATED OBJECTIVE OF CARE

Actual Nursing Problem for Mother and Baby

....

....

....

....

....

Potential Nursing Problems for Mother and Baby

....

....

....

....

NURSING CARE PLAN

ASSESSMENT	NSG DIAGNOSIS	GOAL	PLANNING	IMPLEMENTATION

Health Education to Mother

....

....

....

....

....

....

POSTNATAL AND NEONATAL CARE STUDY

IDENTIFICATION DATA

Name of Mother:...
W/o: ....
Age:...
Ward Name/Bed Number:...
Address: ....
Date of Admission:...
Date of Discharge:...
Obstetrical History – GPLA: ....

PAST MENSTRUAL HISTORY

LMP .... EDD .... Cycle..

HEALTH HISTORY

1. Past Obstetrical History...
....
....
2. Present Pregnancy History
    - I-trimester ....
    ....
    ....
    - II-trimester ....
    ....
    ....
    - III-trimester ....
    ....
    ....
3. Past Medical History ....
....
....
4. Present Surgical History. ....
....
....
5. Past Surgical History. ....
....
....

6. Family History. ....
....
....

7. Personal History. ....
....
....

OBSTETRICAL HISTORY

S.No.	Year	Abortion	Prem	FT	Type of labour and mode of delivery	Gender	Live or Still Birth	Remark

LAB -INVESTIGATION

Hb	Blood Grouping	Blood Sugar	Urine		HIV	VDRL	Any Other
			Albumin	Sugar			

THE PUERPERIUM

Admitted to Postnatal Ward at AM/PM On:

POSTNATAL OBSERVATION CHART FOR MOTHER

Date	Day	Weight	Temp	Pulse	Resp	Fundal Height	Bowel	Urine	Lochia	Breast	Episiotomy Wound	Homen-sign

DELIVERY/OPERATION NOTES

Normal Vaginal Delivery

Type of labour : Spont /induced ....

Mode of delivery: Normal ....

Instrumental ....

Forcep/Vaccum ....

Indication: ....

Operation notes ....

....

....

....

....

....

....

CAESAREAN SECTION

Elective /Emergency..

Indication ....

Type: Lower Segment/Classical ....

Anaesthesia: Ga/Spinal/Epidural ....

Surgical Note..

1st Stage:..............................Hrs...Mins.

2nd Stage:.............................Hrs...Mins.

3rd Stage:.............................Hrs...Mins.

Total : ....Hrs...Mins.

NEWBORN ASSESSMENT

Name of Baby.. Gender.................................. Age...........

Apgar Score .... 1min .... 5 min Condition: Poor/Fair/Good

OBSERVATION CHART-BABY						
Date						
Day						
Weight						
Skin Colour						
Cord						
Eyes						
Mouth						
Urine						
Meconium						
Feeds						
Temperature						
Heart Rate						
Respiration						

Measurement:

Length ....cm

Head Circumference..........cm

Chest Circumference..........cm

Abdominal Circumference..........cm

Reflexes:

Moro: ....

Sucking: ....

Swallowing: ....

Rooting:..........

Grasping: ....

Vaccination: Age of the Baby..........

BCG-Yes/No..........

OPV-Yes/No..........

Hep B-Yes/No ....

NURSING PROBLEMS AND RELATED OBJECTIVE OF CARE

Actual Nursing Problem for Mother and Baby

....

....

....

....

....

Potential Nursing Problems for Mother and Baby

....

....

....

....

NURSING CARE PLAN

ASSESSMENT	NSG DIAGNOSIS	GOAL	PLANNING	IMPLEMENTATION

Health Education to Mother

....

....

....

....

....

....

POSTNATAL AND NEONATAL CARE STUDY

IDENTIFICATION DATA

Name of Mother:..
W/o:..
Age:..
Ward Name/Bed Number:..
Address:..
Date of Admission:..
Date of Discharge:..
Obstetrical History – GPLA:..

PAST MENSTRUAL HISTORY

LMP ....EDD ....Cycle....................................

HEALTH HISTORY

1. Past Obstetrical History..
....
....
2. Present Pregnancy History
   - I-trimester..
   ....
   ....
   - II-trimester..
   ....
   ....
   - III-trimester..
   ....
   ....
3. Past Medical History..
....
....
4. Present Surgical History...
....
....
5. Past Surgical History...
....
....

6. Family History. ....
....
....

7. Personal History. ....
....
....

OBSTETRICAL HISTORY

S.No.	Year	Abortion	Prem	FT	Type of labour and mode of delivery	Gender	Live or Still Birth	Remark

LAB -INVESTIGATION

Hb	Blood Grouping	Blood Sugar	Urine		HIV	VDRL	Any Other
			Albumin	Sugar			

THE PUERPERIUM

Admitted to Postnatal Ward at AM/PM On:

POSTNATAL OBSERVATION CHART FOR MOTHER

Date	Day	Weight	Temp	Pulse	Resp	Fundal Height	Bowel	Urine	Lochia	Breast	Episiotomy Wound	Homen-sign

DELIVERY/OPERATION NOTES

Normal Vaginal Delivery

Type of labour : Spont /induced ....

Mode of delivery: Normal ....

Instrumental ....

Forcep/Vaccum ....

Indication: ....

Operation notes ....

....

....

....

....

....

....

CAESAREAN SECTION

Elective /Emergency..

Indication ....

Type: Lower Segment/Classical ....

Anaesthesia: Ga/Spinal/Epidural ....

Surgical Note..

1st Stage:.............................Hrs...Mins.

2nd Stage:............................Hrs...Mins.

3rd Stage:.............................Hrs...Mins.

Total : ....Hrs...Mins.

NEWBORN ASSESSMENT

Name of Baby... Gender.................................... Age...........

Apgar Score .... 1min ....5 min Condition: Poor/Fair/Good

OBSERVATION CHART-BABY						
Date						
Day						
Weight						
Skin Colour						
Cord						
Eyes						
Mouth						
Urine						
Meconium						
Feeds						
Temperature						
Heart Rate						
Respiration						

Measurement:

Length ....cm

Head Circumference...cm

Chest Circumference..cm

Abdominal Circumference..cm

Reflexes:

Moro: ....

Sucking: ....

Swallowing: ....

Rooting:...

Grasping: ....

Vaccination: Age of the Baby...

BCG-Yes/No...

OPV-Yes/No...

Hep B-Yes/No ....

NURSING PROBLEMS AND RELATED OBJECTIVE OF CARE

Actual Nursing Problem for Mother and Baby

....

....

....

....

....

Potential Nursing Problems for Mother and Baby

....

....

....

....

NURSING CARE PLAN

ASSESSMENT	NSG DIAGNOSIS	GOAL	PLANNING	IMPLEMENTATION

Health Education to Mother

....

....

....

....

....

....

POSTNATAL AND NEONATAL CARE STUDY

IDENTIFICATION DATA

Name of Mother:..

W/o: ....

Age:..

Ward Name/Bed Number:..

Address: ....

Date of Admission:..

Date of Discharge:..

Obstetrical History – GPLA: ....

PAST MENSTRUAL HISTORY

LMP ....EDD ....Cycle..

HEALTH HISTORY

1. Past Obstetrical History..
....
....
2. Present Pregnancy History
   - I-trimester ....
   ....
   ....
   - II-trimester ....
   ....
   ....
   - III-trimester..
   ....
   ....
3. Past Medical History ....
....
....
4. Present Surgical History. ....
....
....
5. Past Surgical History. ....
....
....

6. Family History. ....
....
....
7. Personal History. ....
....
....

OBSTETRICAL HISTORY

S.No.	Year	Abortion	Prem	FT	Type of labour and mode of delivery	Gender	Live or Still Birth	Remark

LAB -INVESTIGATION

Hb	Blood Grouping	Blood Sugar	Urine		HIV	VDRL	Any Other
			Albumin	Sugar			

THE PUERPERIUM

Admitted to Postnatal Ward at AM/PM On:

POSTNATAL OBSERVATION CHART FOR MOTHER

Date	Day	Weight	Temp	Pulse	Resp	Fundal Height	Bowel	Urine	Lochia	Breast	Episiotomy Wound	Homen-sign

DELIVERY/OPERATION NOTES

Normal Vaginal Delivery

Type of labour : Spont /induced ....

Mode of delivery: Normal ....

Instrumental ....

Forcep/Vaccum ....

Indication: ....

Operation notes ....

....

....

....

....

....

....

CAESAREAN SECTION

Elective /Emergency...

Indication ....

Type: Lower Segment/Classical ....

Anaesthesia: Ga/Spinal/Epidural ....

Surgical Note...

1st Stage:...............................Hrs...Mins.

2nd Stage:.............................Hrs...Mins.

3rd Stage: ....Hrs...Mins.

Total : ....Hrs...Mins.

NEWBORN ASSESSMENT

Name of Baby.. Gender.................................... Age...........

Apgar Score .... 1min ....5 min Condition: Poor/Fair/Good

OBSERVATION CHART-BABY						
Date						
Day						
Weight						
Skin Colour						
Cord						
Eyes						
Mouth						
Urine						
Meconium						
Feeds						
Temperature						
Heart Rate						
Respiration						

Measurement:

Length ....cm

Head Circumference..cm

Chest Circumference..cm

Abdominal Circumference..cm

Reflexes:

Moro: ....

Sucking: ....

Swallowing: ....

Rooting:...

Grasping: ....

Vaccination: Age of the Baby...

BCG-Yes/No...

OPV-Yes/No...

Hep B-Yes/No ....

NURSING PROBLEMS AND RELATED OBJECTIVE OF CARE

Actual Nursing Problem for Mother and Baby

....

....

....

....

....

Potential Nursing Problems for Mother and Baby

....

....

....

....

NURSING CARE PLAN

ASSESSMENT	NSG DIAGNOSIS	GOAL	PLANNING	IMPLEMENTATION

Health Education to Mother

....

....

....

....

....

....

POSTNATAL AND NEONATAL CARE STUDY

IDENTIFICATION DATA

Name of Mother:..
W/o: ....
Age:..
Ward Name/Bed Number:..
Address: ....
Date of Admission:..
Date of Discharge:..
Obstetrical History – GPLA: ....

PAST MENSTRUAL HISTORY

LMP .... EDD .... Cycle..

HEALTH HISTORY

1. Past Obstetrical History..
   ....
   ....
2. Present Pregnancy History
   - I-trimester ....
     ....
     ....
   - II-trimester ....
     ....
     ....
   - III-trimester..
     ....
     ....
3. Past Medical History ....
   ....
   ....
4. Present Surgical History. ....
   ....
   ....
5. Past Surgical History. ....
   ....
   ....

6. Family History. ....
....
....

7. Personal History. ....
....
....

OBSTETRICAL HISTORY

S.No.	Year	Abortion	Prem	FT	Type of labour and mode of delivery	Gender	Live or Still Birth	Remark

LAB -INVESTIGATION

Hb	Blood Grouping	Blood Sugar	Urine		HIV	VDRL	Any Other
			Albumin	Sugar			

THE PUERPERIUM

Admitted to Postnatal Ward at AM/PM On:

POSTNATAL OBSERVATION CHART FOR MOTHER

Date	Day	Weight	Temp	Pulse	Resp	Fundal Height	Bowel	Urine	Lochia	Breast	Episiotomy Wound	Homen-sign

DELIVERY/OPERATION NOTES

Normal Vaginal Delivery

Type of labour : Spont /induced ....

Mode of delivery: Normal ....

Instrumental ....

Forcep/Vaccum ....

Indication: ....

Operation notes ....

....

....

....

....

....

....

CAESAREAN SECTION

Elective /Emergency...

Indication ....

Type: Lower Segment/Classical ....

Anaesthesia: Ga/Spinal/Epidural ....

Surgical Note...

1st Stage:...............................Hrs..Mins.

2nd Stage:.............................Hrs..Mins.

3rd Stage:..............................Hrs..Mins.

Total : ....Hrs..Mins.

NEWBORN ASSESSMENT

Name of Baby..Gender.................................... Age...........

Apgar Score .... 1min .... 5 min Condition: Poor/Fair/Good

OBSERVATION CHART-BABY						
Date						
Day						
Weight						
Skin Colour						
Cord						
Eyes						
Mouth						
Urine						
Meconium						
Feeds						
Temperature						
Heart Rate						
Respiration						

Measurement:

Length ....cm

Head Circumference...cm

Chest Circumference..cm

Abdominal Circumference..cm

Reflexes:

Moro: ....

Sucking: ....

Swallowing: ....

Rooting:...

Grasping: ....

Vaccination: Age of the Baby...

BCG-Yes/No...

OPV-Yes/No...

Hep B-Yes/No ....

NURSING PROBLEMS AND RELATED OBJECTIVE OF CARE

Actual Nursing Problem for Mother and Baby

....

....

....

....

....

Potential Nursing Problems for Mother and Baby

....

....

....

....

NURSING CARE PLAN

ASSESSMENT	NSG DIAGNOSIS	GOAL	PLANNING	IMPLEMENTATION

Health Education to Mother

....

....

....

....

....

....

POSTNATAL AND NEONATAL CARE STUDY

IDENTIFICATION DATA

Name of Mother:..
W/o: ....
Age:..
Ward Name/Bed Number:..
Address: ....
Date of Admission:...
Date of Discharge:..
Obstetrical History – GPLA: ....

PAST MENSTRUAL HISTORY

LMP ....EDD ....Cycle...

HEALTH HISTORY

1. Past Obstetrical History..
   ....
   ....
2. Present Pregnancy History
   - I-trimester ....
     ....
     ....
   - II-trimester ....
     ....
     ....
   - III-trimester...
     ....
     ....
3. Past Medical History ....
   ....
   ....
4. Present Surgical History. ....
   ....
   ....
5. Past Surgical History. ....
   ....
   ....

6. Family History. ....
....
....

7. Personal History. ....
....
....

OBSTETRICAL HISTORY

S.No.	Year	Abortion	Prem	FT	Type of labour and mode of delivery	Gender	Live or Still Birth	Remark

LAB -INVESTIGATION

Hb	Blood Grouping	Blood Sugar	Urine		HIV	VDRL	Any Other
			Albumin	Sugar			

THE PUERPERIUM

Admitted to Postnatal Ward at AM/PM On:

POSTNATAL OBSERVATION CHART FOR MOTHER

Date	Day	Weight	Temp	Pulse	Resp	Fundal Height	Bowel	Urine	Lochia	Breast	Episiotomy Wound	Homen-sign

DELIVERY/OPERATION NOTES

Normal Vaginal Delivery

Type of labour : Spont /induced ....

Mode of delivery: Normal ....

Instrumental ....

Forcep/Vaccum ....

Indication: ....

Operation notes ....

....

....

....

....

....

....

CAESAREAN SECTION

Elective /Emergency..

Indication ....

Type: Lower Segment/Classical ....

Anaesthesia: Ga/Spinal/Epidural ....

Surgical Note..

1st Stage:..............................Hrs...Mins.

2nd Stage:............................Hrs...Mins.

3rd Stage: ....Hrs...Mins.

Total : ....Hrs...Mins.

NEWBORN ASSESSMENT

Name of Baby.. Gender.................................. Age...........

Apgar Score .... 1min ....5 min Condition: Poor/Fair/Good

OBSERVATION CHART-BABY						
Date						
Day						
Weight						
Skin Colour						
Cord						
Eyes						
Mouth						
Urine						
Meconium						
Feeds						
Temperature						
Heart Rate						
Respiration						

Measurement:

Length ....cm

Head Circumference..cm

Chest Circumference..cm

Abdominal Circumference...cm

Reflexes:

Moro: ....

Sucking: ....

Swallowing: ....

Rooting:..

Grasping: ....

Vaccination: Age of the Baby...

BCG-Yes/No...

OPV-Yes/No...

Hep B-Yes/No ....

NURSING PROBLEMS AND RELATED OBJECTIVE OF CARE

Actual Nursing Problem for Mother and Baby

....

....

....

....

....

Potential Nursing Problems for Mother and Baby

....

....

....

....

NURSING CARE PLAN

ASSESSMENT	NSG DIAGNOSIS	GOAL	PLANNING	IMPLEMENTATION

Health Education to Mother

....

....

....

....

....

....

POSTNATAL AND NEONATAL CARE STUDY

IDENTIFICATION DATA

Name of Mother:...

W/o:...

Age:...

Ward Name/Bed Number:...

Address:...

Date of Admission:...

Date of Discharge:...

Obstetrical History – GPLA:...

PAST MENSTRUAL HISTORY

LMP ....EDD ....Cycle...

HEALTH HISTORY

1. Past Obstetrical History...

   ....

   ....

2. Present Pregnancy History

   - I-trimester...

     ....

     ....

   - II-trimester...

     ....

     ....

   - III-trimester...

     ....

     ....

3. Past Medical History...

   ....

   ....

4. Present Surgical History...

   ....

   ....

5. Past Surgical History...

   ....

   ....

6. Family History. ....
....
....

7. Personal History. ....
....
....

OBSTETRICAL HISTORY

S.No.	Year	Abortion	Prem	FT	Type of labour and mode of delivery	Gender	Live or Still Birth	Remark

LAB -INVESTIGATION

Hb	Blood Grouping	Blood Sugar	Urine		HIV	VDRL	Any Other
			Albumin	Sugar			

THE PUERPERIUM

Admitted to Postnatal Ward at AM/PM On:

POSTNATAL OBSERVATION CHART FOR MOTHER

Date	Day	Weight	Temp	Pulse	Resp	Fundal Height	Bowel	Urine	Lochia	Breast	Episiotomy Wound	Homen-sign

DELIVERY/OPERATION NOTES

Normal Vaginal Delivery

Type of labour : Spont /induced ....

Mode of delivery: Normal ....

Instrumental ....

Forcep/Vaccum ....

Indication: ....

Operation notes ....

....

....

....

....

....

....

CAESAREAN SECTION

Elective /Emergency...

Indication ....

Type: Lower Segment/Classical ....

Anaesthesia: Ga/Spinal/Epidural ....

Surgical Note...

1st Stage:................................Hrs...Mins.

2nd Stage:..............................Hrs...Mins.

3rd Stage:..............................Hrs...Mins.

Total :.....................................Hrs...Mins.

NEWBORN ASSESSMENT

Name of Baby.. Gender.................................... Age...........

Apgar Score .... 1min ....5 min Condition: Poor/Fair/Good

OBSERVATION CHART-BABY						
Date						
Day						
Weight						
Skin Colour						
Cord						
Eyes						
Mouth						
Urine						
Meconium						
Feeds						
Temperature						
Heart Rate						
Respiration						

Measurement:

Length ....cm

Head Circumference...cm

Chest Circumference..cm

Abdominal Circumference...cm

Reflexes:

Moro: ....

Sucking: ....

Swallowing: ....

Rooting:..

Grasping: ....

Vaccination: Age of the Baby...

BCG-Yes/No...

OPV-Yes/No...

Hep B-Yes/No ....

NURSING PROBLEMS AND RELATED OBJECTIVE OF CARE

Actual Nursing Problem for Mother and Baby

....

....

....

....

....

Potential Nursing Problems for Mother and Baby

....

....

....

....

NURSING CARE PLAN

ASSESSMENT	NSG DIAGNOSIS	GOAL	PLANNING	IMPLEMENTATION

Health Education to Mother

....

....

....

....

....

....

POSTNATAL AND NEONATAL CARE STUDY

IDENTIFICATION DATA

Name of Mother:..

W/o:..

Age:..

Ward Name/Bed Number:..

Address:..

Date of Admission:..

Date of Discharge:..

Obstetrical History – GPLA:..

PAST MENSTRUAL HISTORY

LMP .... EDD .... Cycle ....

HEALTH HISTORY

1. Past Obstetrical History..
....
....

2. Present Pregnancy History
   - I-trimester..
     ....
     ....
   - II-trimester..
     ....
     ....
   - III-trimester..
     ....
     ....

3. Past Medical History..
....
....

4. Present Surgical History...
....
....

5. Past Surgical History...
....
....

6. Family History. ....

....

....

7. Personal History. ....

....

....

OBSTETRICAL HISTORY

S.No.	Year	Abortion	Prem	FT	Type of labour and mode of delivery	Gender	Live or Still Birth	Remark

LAB -INVESTIGATION

Hb	Blood Grouping	Blood Sugar	Urine		HIV	VDRL	Any Other
			Albumin	Sugar			

THE PUERPERIUM

Admitted to Postnatal Ward at AM/PM On:

POSTNATAL OBSERVATION CHART FOR MOTHER

Date	Day	Weight	Temp	Pulse	Resp	Fundal Height	Bowel	Urine	Lochia	Breast	Episiotomy Wound	Homen-sign

DELIVERY/OPERATION NOTES

Normal Vaginal Delivery

Type of labour : Spont /induced ....

Mode of delivery: Normal ....

Instrumental ....

Forcep/Vaccum ....

Indication: ....

Operation notes ....

....

....

....

....

....

....

CAESAREAN SECTION

Elective /Emergency..

Indication ....

Type: Lower Segment/Classical ....

Anaesthesia: Ga/Spinal/Epidural ....

Surgical Note..

1st Stage:..............................Hrs...Mins.

2nd Stage:.............................Hrs...Mins.

3rd Stage: ....Hrs...Mins.

Total : ....Hrs...Mins.

NEWBORN ASSESSMENT

Name of Baby... Gender.................................. Age...........

Apgar Score .... 1min ....5 min Condition: Poor/Fair/Good

OBSERVATION CHART-BABY						
Date						
Day						
Weight						
Skin Colour						
Cord						
Eyes						
Mouth						
Urine						
Meconium						
Feeds						
Temperature						
Heart Rate						
Respiration						

Measurement:

Length ....cm

Head Circumference..cm

Chest Circumference..cm

Abdominal Circumference...cm

Reflexes:

Moro: ....

Sucking: ....

Swallowing: ....

Rooting:...

Grasping: ....

Vaccination: Age of the Baby...

BCG-Yes/No...

OPV-Yes/No...

Hep B-Yes/No ....

NURSING PROBLEMS AND RELATED OBJECTIVE OF CARE

Actual Nursing Problem for Mother and Baby

....

....

....

....

....

Potential Nursing Problems for Mother and Baby

....

....

....

....

NURSING CARE PLAN

ASSESSMENT	NSG DIAGNOSIS	GOAL	PLANNING	IMPLEMENTATION

Health Education to Mother

....

....

....

....

....

....

POSTNATAL AND NEONATAL CARE STUDY

IDENTIFICATION DATA

Name of Mother:..

W/o: ....

Age:..

Ward Name/Bed Number:..

Address: ....

Date of Admission:..

Date of Discharge:..

Obstetrical History – GPLA: ....

PAST MENSTRUAL HISTORY

LMP ....EDD ....Cycle..

HEALTH HISTORY

1. Past Obstetrical History..

   ....

   ....

2. Present Pregnancy History
   - I-trimester ....

     ....

     ....
   - II-trimester..

     ....

     ....
   - III-trimester..

     ....

     ....
3. Past Medical History ....

   ....

   ....
4. Present Surgical History. ....

   ....

   ....
5. Past Surgical History. ....

   ....

   ....

6. Family History. ....
....
....

7. Personal History. ....
....
....

OBSTETRICAL HISTORY

S.No.	Year	Abortion	Prem	FT	Type of labour and mode of delivery	Gender	Live or Still Birth	Remark

LAB -INVESTIGATION

Hb	Blood Grouping	Blood Sugar	Urine		HIV	VDRL	Any Other
			Albumin	Sugar			

THE PUERPERIUM

Admitted to Postnatal Ward at AM/PM On:

POSTNATAL OBSERVATION CHART FOR MOTHER

Date	Day	Weight	Temp	Pulse	Resp	Fundal Height	Bowel	Urine	Lochia	Breast	Episiotomy Wound	Homen-sign

DELIVERY/OPERATION NOTES

Normal Vaginal Delivery

Type of labour : Spont /induced ....

Mode of delivery: Normal ....

Instrumental ....

Forcep/Vaccum ....

Indication: ....

Operation notes ....

....

....

....

....

....

....

CAESAREAN SECTION

Elective /Emergency...

Indication ....

Type: Lower Segment/Classical ....

Anaesthesia: Ga/Spinal/Epidural ....

Surgical Note...

1st Stage:...............................Hrs...Mins.

2nd Stage:.............................Hrs...Mins.

3rd Stage:.............................Hrs...Mins.

Total : ....Hrs...Mins.

NEWBORN ASSESSMENT

Name of Baby... Gender.................................. Age...........

Apgar Score .... 1min ....5 min Condition: Poor/Fair/Good

OBSERVATION CHART-BABY						
Date						
Day						
Weight						
Skin Colour						
Cord						
Eyes						
Mouth						
Urine						
Meconium						
Feeds						
Temperature						
Heart Rate						
Respiration						

Measurement:

Length ....cm

Head Circumference..cm

Chest Circumference..cm

Abdominal Circumference..cm

Reflexes:

Moro: ....

Sucking: ....

Swallowing: ....

Rooting:..

Grasping: ....

Vaccination: Age of the Baby..

BCG-Yes/No...

OPV-Yes/No...

Hep B-Yes/No ....

NURSING PROBLEMS AND RELATED OBJECTIVE OF CARE

Actual Nursing Problem for Mother and Baby

....

....

....

....

....

Potential Nursing Problems for Mother and Baby

....

....

....

....

NURSING CARE PLAN

ASSESSMENT	NSG DIAGNOSIS	GOAL	PLANNING	IMPLEMENTATION

Health Education to Mother

....

....

....

....

....

....

POSTNATAL AND NEONATAL CARE STUDY

IDENTIFICATION DATA

Name of Mother:..

W/o: ....

Age:..

Ward Name/Bed Number:..

Address: ....

Date of Admission:..

Date of Discharge:..

Obstetrical History – GPLA: ....

PAST MENSTRUAL HISTORY

LMP ....EDD ....Cycle...

HEALTH HISTORY

1. Past Obstetrical History..
 ....
 ....
2. Present Pregnancy History
 - I-trimester..
 ....
 ....
 - II-trimester..
 ....
 ....
 - III-trimester..
 ....
 ....
3. Past Medical History..
 ....
 ....
4. Present Surgical History. ....
 ....
 ....
5. Past Surgical History. ....
 ....
 ....

6. Family History. ....

....

....

7. Personal History. ....

....

....

OBSTETRICAL HISTORY

S.No.	Year	Abortion	Prem	FT	Type of labour and mode of delivery	Gender	Live or Still Birth	Remark

LAB -INVESTIGATION

Hb	Blood Grouping	Blood Sugar	Urine		HIV	VDRL	Any Other
			Albumin	Sugar			

THE PUERPERIUM

Admitted to Postnatal Ward at AM/PM On:

POSTNATAL OBSERVATION CHART FOR MOTHER

Date	Day	Weight	Temp	Pulse	Resp	Fundal Height	Bowel	Urine	Lochia	Breast	Episiotomy Wound	Homen-sign

DELIVERY/OPERATION NOTES

Normal Vaginal Delivery

Type of labour : Spont /induced ....

Mode of delivery: Normal ....

Instrumental ....

Forcep/Vaccum ....

Indication: ....

Operation notes ....

....

....

....

....

....

....

CAESAREAN SECTION

Elective /Emergency..

Indication ....

Type: Lower Segment/Classical ....

Anaesthesia: Ga/Spinal/Epidural ....

Surgical Note..

1st Stage:..............................Hrs..Mins.

2nd Stage:.............................Hrs..Mins.

3rd Stage:..............................Hrs..Mins.

Total : ....Hrs..Mins.

NEWBORN ASSESSMENT

Name of Baby.. Gender.................................. Age...........

Apgar Score .... 1min ....5 min Condition: Poor/Fair/Good

OBSERVATION CHART-BABY						
Date						
Day						
Weight						
Skin Colour						
Cord						
Eyes						
Mouth						
Urine						
Meconium						
Feeds						
Temperature						
Heart Rate						
Respiration						

Measurement:

Length ....cm

Head Circumference..cm

Chest Circumference..cm

Abdominal Circumference..cm

Reflexes:

Moro: ....

Sucking: ....

Swallowing: ....

Rooting:...

Grasping: ....

Vaccination: Age of the Baby...

BCG-Yes/No...

OPV-Yes/No...

Hep B-Yes/No ....

NURSING PROBLEMS AND RELATED OBJECTIVE OF CARE

Actual Nursing Problem for Mother and Baby

....

....

....

....

....

Potential Nursing Problems for Mother and Baby

....

....

....

....

NURSING CARE PLAN

ASSESSMENT	NSG DIAGNOSIS	GOAL	PLANNING	IMPLEMENTATION

Health Education to Mother

....

....

....

....

....

....

POSTNATAL AND NEONATAL CARE STUDY

IDENTIFICATION DATA

Name of Mother:...

W/o: ....

Age:...

Ward Name/Bed Number:...

Address: ....

Date of Admission:...

Date of Discharge:...

Obstetrical History – GPLA: ....

PAST MENSTRUAL HISTORY

LMP ....EDD ....Cycle..................................

HEALTH HISTORY

1. Past Obstetrical History...
   ....
   ....
2. Present Pregnancy History
   - I-trimester ....
     ....
     ....
   - II-trimester...
     ....
     ....
   - III-trimester...
     ....
     ....
3. Past Medical History ....
   ....
   ....
4. Present Surgical History. ....
   ....
   ....
5. Past Surgical History. ....
   ....
   ....

6. Family History. ....
....
....

7. Personal History. ....
....
....

OBSTETRICAL HISTORY

S.No.	Year	Abortion	Prem	FT	Type of labour and mode of delivery	Gender	Live or Still Birth	Remark

LAB -INVESTIGATION

Hb	Blood Grouping	Blood Sugar	Urine		HIV	VDRL	Any Other
			Albumin	Sugar			

THE PUERPERIUM

Admitted to Postnatal Ward at AM/PM On:

POSTNATAL OBSERVATION CHART FOR MOTHER

Date	Day	Weight	Temp	Pulse	Resp	Fundal Height	Bowel	Urine	Lochia	Breast	Episiotomy Wound	Homen-sign

DELIVERY/OPERATION NOTES

Normal Vaginal Delivery

Type of labour : Spont /induced ....

Mode of delivery: Normal ....

Instrumental ....

Forcep/Vaccum..

Indication:..

Operation notes ....

....

....

....

....

....

....

CAESAREAN SECTION

Elective /Emergency..

Indication ....

Type: Lower Segment/Classical ....

Anaesthesia: Ga/Spinal/Epidural ....

Surgical Note...

1st Stage:..............................Hrs..Mins.

2nd Stage:............................Hrs..Mins.

3rd Stage:.............................Hrs..Mins.

Total : ....Hrs..Mins.

NEWBORN ASSESSMENT

Name of Baby... Gender.................................... Age...........

Apgar Score .... 1min ....5 min Condition: Poor/Fair/Good

OBSERVATION CHART-BABY						
Date						
Day						
Weight						
Skin Colour						
Cord						
Eyes						
Mouth						
Urine						
Meconium						
Feeds						
Temperature						
Heart Rate						
Respiration						

Measurement:

Length ....cm

Head Circumference..cm

Chest Circumference...cm

Abdominal Circumference..cm

Reflexes:

Moro: ....

Sucking: ....

Swallowing: ....

Rooting:...

Grasping: ....

Vaccination: Age of the Baby...

BCG-Yes/No...

OPV-Yes/No...

Hep B-Yes/No ....

NURSING PROBLEMS AND RELATED OBJECTIVE OF CARE

Actual Nursing Problem for Mother and Baby

....

....

....

....

....

Potential Nursing Problems for Mother and Baby

....

....

....

....

NURSING CARE PLAN

ASSESSMENT	NSG DIAGNOSIS	GOAL	PLANNING	IMPLEMENTATION

Health Education to Mother

....

....

....

....

....

....

POSTNATAL AND NEONATAL CARE STUDY

IDENTIFICATION DATA

Name of Mother:...

W/o: ....

Age:...

Ward Name/Bed Number:...

Address: ....

Date of Admission:..

Date of Discharge:...

Obstetrical History – GPLA: ....

PAST MENSTRUAL HISTORY

LMP ....EDD ....Cycle..

HEALTH HISTORY

1. Past Obstetrical History..
   ....
   ....
2. Present Pregnancy History
   - I-trimester ....
     ....
     ....
   - II-trimester ....
     ....
     ....
   - III-trimester ....
     ....
     ....
3. Past Medical History ....
   ....
   ....
4. Present Surgical History. ....
   ....
   ....
5. Past Surgical History. ....
   ....
   ....

6. Family History. ....
....
....

7. Personal History. ....
....
....

OBSTETRICAL HISTORY

S.No.	Year	Abortion	Prem	FT	Type of labour and mode of delivery	Gender	Live or Still Birth	Remark

LAB -INVESTIGATION

Hb	Blood Grouping	Blood Sugar	Urine		HIV	VDRL	Any Other
			Albumin	Sugar			

THE PUERPERIUM

Admitted to Postnatal Ward at AM/PM On:

POSTNATAL OBSERVATION CHART FOR MOTHER

Date	Day	Weight	Temp	Pulse	Resp	Fundal Height	Bowel	Urine	Lochia	Breast	Episiotomy Wound	Homen-sign

DELIVERY/OPERATION NOTES

Normal Vaginal Delivery

Type of labour : Spont /induced ....

Mode of delivery: Normal ....

Instrumental ....

Forcep/Vaccum ....

Indication: ....

Operation notes ....

....

....

....

....

....

....

CAESAREAN SECTION

Elective /Emergency..

Indication ....

Type: Lower Segment/Classical ....

Anaesthesia: Ga/Spinal/Epidural ....

Surgical Note..

1st Stage:...............................Hrs...Mins.

2nd Stage:.............................Hrs...Mins.

3rd Stage: ....Hrs...Mins.

Total : ....Hrs...Mins.

NEWBORN ASSESSMENT

Name of Baby...Gender.................................... Age...........

Apgar Score .... 1min ....5 min Condition: Poor/Fair/Good

OBSERVATION CHART-BABY						
Date						
Day						
Weight						
Skin Colour						
Cord						
Eyes						
Mouth						
Urine						
Meconium						
Feeds						
Temperature						
Heart Rate						
Respiration						

Measurement:

Length ....cm

Head Circumference...cm

Chest Circumference...cm

Abdominal Circumference...cm

Reflexes:

Moro: ....

Sucking: ....

Swallowing: ....

Rooting:...

Grasping: ....

Vaccination: Age of the Baby...

BCG-Yes/No..

OPV-Yes/No..

Hep B-Yes/No ....

NURSING PROBLEMS AND RELATED OBJECTIVE OF CARE

Actual Nursing Problem for Mother and Baby

....

....

....

....

....

Potential Nursing Problems for Mother and Baby

....

....

....

....

NURSING CARE PLAN

ASSESSMENT	NSG DIAGNOSIS	GOAL	PLANNING	IMPLEMENTATION

Health Education to Mother

....

....

....

....

....

....

POSTNATAL AND NEONATAL CARE STUDY

IDENTIFICATION DATA

Name of Mother:...

W/o: ....

Age:...

Ward Name/Bed Number:...

Address: ....

Date of Admission:...

Date of Discharge:...

Obstetrical History – GPLA: ....

PAST MENSTRUAL HISTORY

LMP ....EDD ....Cycle..

HEALTH HISTORY

1. Past Obstetrical History...
....
....
2. Present Pregnancy History
   - I-trimester...
   ....
   ....
   - II-trimester...
   ....
   ....
   - III-trimester...
   ....
   ....
3. Past Medical History...
....
....
4. Present Surgical History. ....
....
....
5. Past Surgical History. ....
....
....

6. Family History. ....
....
....

7. Personal History. ....
....
....

OBSTETRICAL HISTORY

S.No.	Year	Abortion	Prem	FT	Type of labour and mode of delivery	Gender	Live or Still Birth	Remark

LAB -INVESTIGATION

Hb	Blood Grouping	Blood Sugar	Urine		HIV	VDRL	Any Other
			Albumin	Sugar			

THE PUERPERIUM

Admitted to Postnatal Ward at AM/PM On:

POSTNATAL OBSERVATION CHART FOR MOTHER

Date	Day	Weight	Temp	Pulse	Resp	Fundal Height	Bowel	Urine	Lochia	Breast	Episiotomy Wound	Homen-sign

DELIVERY/OPERATION NOTES

Normal Vaginal Delivery

Type of labour : Spont /induced ....

Mode of delivery: Normal..

Instrumental..

Forcep/Vaccum..

Indication:..

Operation notes ....

....

....

....

....

....

....

CAESAREAN SECTION

Elective /Emergency...

Indication ....

Type: Lower Segment/Classical ....

Anaesthesia: Ga/Spinal/Epidural ....

Surgical Note...

1st Stage:.............................Hrs...Mins.

2nd Stage:...........................Hrs...Mins.

3rd Stage: ....Hrs...Mins.

Total : ....Hrs...Mins.

NEWBORN ASSESSMENT

Name of Baby..Gender.................................... Age...........

Apgar Score ....1min ....5 min Condition: Poor/Fair/Good

OBSERVATION CHART-BABY						
Date						
Day						
Weight						
Skin Colour						
Cord						
Eyes						
Mouth						
Urine						
Meconium						
Feeds						
Temperature						
Heart Rate						
Respiration						

Measurement:

Length ....cm

Head Circumference..cm

Chest Circumference...cm

Abdominal Circumference....................................cm

Reflexes:

Moro: ....

Sucking: ....

Swallowing: ....

Rooting:...

Grasping: ....

Vaccination: Age of the Baby...

BCG-Yes/No..

OPV-Yes/No..

Hep B-Yes/No ....

NURSING PROBLEMS AND RELATED OBJECTIVE OF CARE

Actual Nursing Problem for Mother and Baby

....

....

....

....

....

Potential Nursing Problems for Mother and Baby

....

....

....

....

NURSING CARE PLAN

ASSESSMENT	NSG DIAGNOSIS	GOAL	PLANNING	IMPLEMENTATION

Health Education to Mother

....

....

....

....

....

....

POSTNATAL AND NEONATAL CARE STUDY

IDENTIFICATION DATA

Name of Mother:..

W/o:..

Age:..

Ward Name/Bed Number:..

Address:..

Date of Admission:..

Date of Discharge:..

Obstetrical History – GPLA:..

PAST MENSTRUAL HISTORY

LMP .... EDD .... Cycle ....

HEALTH HISTORY

1. Past Obstetrical History..
....
....
2. Present Pregnancy History
   - I-trimester..
     ....
     ....
   - II-trimester..
     ....
     ....
   - III-trimester..
     ....
     ....
3. Past Medical History..
....
....
4. Present Surgical History. ....
....
....
5. Past Surgical History. ....
....
....

6. Family History. ....

....

....

7. Personal History. ....

....

....

OBSTETRICAL HISTORY

S.No.	Year	Abortion	Prem	FT	Type of labour and mode of delivery	Gender	Live or Still Birth	Remark

LAB -INVESTIGATION

Hb	Blood Grouping	Blood Sugar	Urine		HIV	VDRL	Any Other
			Albumin	Sugar			

THE PUERPERIUM

Admitted to Postnatal Ward at AM/PM On:

POSTNATAL OBSERVATION CHART FOR MOTHER

Date	Day	Weight	Temp	Pulse	Resp	Fundal Height	Bowel	Urine	Lochia	Breast	Episiotomy Wound	Homen-sign

DELIVERY/OPERATION NOTES

Normal Vaginal Delivery

Type of labour : Spont /induced ....

Mode of delivery: Normal..

Instrumental..

Forcep/Vaccum..

Indication:..

Operation notes ....

....

....

....

....

....

....

CAESAREAN SECTION

Elective /Emergency..

Indication ....

Type: Lower Segment/Classical ....

Anaesthesia: Ga/Spinal/Epidural ....

Surgical Note..

1st Stage:..............................Hrs..Mins.

2nd Stage:............................Hrs..Mins.

3rd Stage: ....Hrs..Mins.

Total : ....Hrs..Mins.

NEWBORN ASSESSMENT

Name of Baby..Gender.................................. Age...........

Apgar Score ....1min ....5 min Condition: Poor/Fair/Good

OBSERVATION CHART-BABY						
Date						
Day						
Weight						
Skin Colour						
Cord						
Eyes						
Mouth						
Urine						
Meconium						
Feeds						
Temperature						
Heart Rate						
Respiration						

Measurement:

Length ....cm

Head Circumference..cm

Chest Circumference ....cm

Abdominal Circumference ....cm

Reflexes:

Moro: ....

Sucking: ....

Swallowing: ....

Rooting:..

Grasping: ....

Vaccination: Age of the Baby...

BCG-Yes/No..

OPV-Yes/No..

Hep B-Yes/No ....

NURSING PROBLEMS AND RELATED OBJECTIVE OF CARE

Actual Nursing Problem for Mother and Baby

....

....

....

....

....

Potential Nursing Problems for Mother and Baby

....

....

....

....

NURSING CARE PLAN

ASSESSMENT	NSG DIAGNOSIS	GOAL	PLANNING	IMPLEMENTATION

Health Education to Mother

....

....

....

....

....

....

POSTNATAL AND NEONATAL CARE STUDY

IDENTIFICATION DATA

Name of Mother:..........

W/o:..........

Age:..........

Ward Name/Bed Number:..........

Address:..........

Date of Admission:..........

Date of Discharge:..........

Obstetrical History – GPLA:..........

PAST MENSTRUAL HISTORY

LMP .... EDD .... Cycle ....

HEALTH HISTORY

1. Past Obstetrical History..........
....
....
2. Present Pregnancy History
   - I-trimester..........
   ....
   ....
   - II-trimester..........
   ....
   ....
   - III-trimester..........
   ....
   ....
3. Past Medical History..........
....
....
4. Present Surgical History...........
....
....
5. Past Surgical History...........
....
....

6. Family History. ....

7. Personal History. ....

OBSTETRICAL HISTORY

S.No.	Year	Abortion	Prem	FT	Type of labour and mode of delivery	Gender	Live or Still Birth	Remark

LAB -INVESTIGATION

Hb	Blood Grouping	Blood Sugar	Urine		HIV	VDRL	Any Other
			Albumin	Sugar			

THE PUERPERIUM

Admitted to Postnatal Ward at AM/PM On:

POSTNATAL OBSERVATION CHART FOR MOTHER

Date	Day	Weight	Temp	Pulse	Resp	Fundal Height	Bowel	Urine	Lochia	Breast	Episiotomy Wound	Homen-sign

DELIVERY/OPERATION NOTES

Normal Vaginal Delivery

Type of labour : Spont /induced ....

Mode of delivery: Normal ....

Instrumental ....

Forcep/Vaccum ....

Indication: ....

Operation notes ....

....

....

....

....

....

....

CAESAREAN SECTION

Elective /Emergency...

Indication ....

Type: Lower Segment/Classical ....

Anaesthesia: Ga/Spinal/Epidural ....

Surgical Note...

1st Stage:..............................Hrs...Mins.

2nd Stage:.............................Hrs...Mins.

3rd Stage:..............................Hrs...Mins.

Total : ....Hrs...Mins.

NEWBORN ASSESSMENT

Name of Baby..Gender..................................... Age...........

Apgar Score ....1min ....5 min Condition: Poor/Fair/Good

OBSERVATION CHART-BABY						
Date						
Day						
Weight						
Skin Colour						
Cord						
Eyes						
Mouth						
Urine						
Meconium						
Feeds						
Temperature						
Heart Rate						
Respiration						

Measurement:

Length ....cm

Head Circumference..cm

Chest Circumference..cm

Abdominal Circumference..cm

Reflexes:

Moro: ....

Sucking: ....

Swallowing: ....

Rooting:...

Grasping: ....

Vaccination: Age of the Baby...

BCG-Yes/No..

OPV-Yes/No...

Hep B-Yes/No ....

NURSING PROBLEMS AND RELATED OBJECTIVE OF CARE

Actual Nursing Problem for Mother and Baby

....

....

....

....

....

Potential Nursing Problems for Mother and Baby

....

....

....

....

NURSING CARE PLAN

ASSESSMENT	NSG DIAGNOSIS	GOAL	PLANNING	IMPLEMENTATION

Health Education to Mother

....

....

....

....

....

....

POSTNATAL AND NEONATAL CARE STUDY

IDENTIFICATION DATA

Name of Mother:..............................

W/o:..............................

Age:..............................

Ward Name/Bed Number:..............................

Address:..............................

Date of Admission:..............................

Date of Discharge:..............................

Obstetrical History – GPLA:..............................

PAST MENSTRUAL HISTORY

LMP .... EDD .... Cycle ....

HEALTH HISTORY

1. Past Obstetrical History..............................
   ....
   ....
2. Present Pregnancy History
   - I-trimester..............................
     ....
     ....
   - II-trimester..............................
     ....
     ....
   - III-trimester..............................
     ....
     ....
3. Past Medical History..............................
   ....
   ....
4. Present Surgical History...............................
   ....
   ....
5. Past Surgical History...............................
   ....
   ....

6. Family History. ....
....
....
7. Personal History. ....
....
....

OBSTETRICAL HISTORY

S.No.	Year	Abortion	Prem	FT	Type of labour and mode of delivery	Gender	Live or Still Birth	Remark

LAB -INVESTIGATION

Hb	Blood Grouping	Blood Sugar	Urine		HIV	VDRL	Any Other
			Albumin	Sugar			

THE PUERPERIUM

Admitted to Postnatal Ward at AM/PM On:

POSTNATAL OBSERVATION CHART FOR MOTHER

Date	Day	Weight	Temp	Pulse	Resp	Fundal Height	Bowel	Urine	Lochia	Breast	Episiotomy Wound	Homen-sign

DELIVERY/OPERATION NOTES

Normal Vaginal Delivery

Type of labour : Spont /induced ....

Mode of delivery: Normal..

Instrumental ....

Forcep/Vaccum..

Indication:..

Operation notes ....

....

....

....

....

....

....

CAESAREAN SECTION

Elective /Emergency...

Indication ....

Type: Lower Segment/Classical ....

Anaesthesia: Ga/Spinal/Epidural ....

Surgical Note...

1st Stage:..............................Hrs...Mins.

2nd Stage:............................Hrs...Mins.

3rd Stage: ....Hrs...Mins.

Total : ....Hrs...Mins.

NEWBORN ASSESSMENT

Name of Baby.. Gender.................................... Age...........

Apgar Score .... 1min ....5 min Condition: Poor/Fair/Good

OBSERVATION CHART-BABY						
Date						
Day						
Weight						
Skin Colour						
Cord						
Eyes						
Mouth						
Urine						
Meconium						
Feeds						
Temperature						
Heart Rate						
Respiration						

Measurement:

Length...cm

Head Circumference...cm

Chest Circumference...cm

Abdominal Circumference...cm

Reflexes:

Moro: ....

Sucking: ....

Swallowing: ....

Rooting:...

Grasping: ....

Vaccination: Age of the Baby...

BCG-Yes/No...

OPV-Yes/No...

Hep B-Yes/No ....

NURSING PROBLEMS AND RELATED OBJECTIVE OF CARE

Actual Nursing Problem for Mother and Baby

....

....

....

....

....

Potential Nursing Problems for Mother and Baby

....

....

....

....

NURSING CARE PLAN

ASSESSMENT	NSG DIAGNOSIS	GOAL	PLANNING	IMPLEMENTATION

Health Education to Mother

....

....

....

....

....

....

POSTNATAL AND NEONATAL CARE STUDY

IDENTIFICATION DATA

Name of Mother:..

W/o: ....

Age:..

Ward Name/Bed Number:...

Address: ....

Date of Admission:...

Date of Discharge:...

Obstetrical History – GPLA: ....

PAST MENSTRUAL HISTORY

LMP ....EDD ....Cycle..

HEALTH HISTORY

1. Past Obstetrical History..
   ....
   ....
2. Present Pregnancy History
   - I-trimester ....
     ....
     ....
   - II-trimester...
     ....
     ....
   - III-trimester..
     ....
     ....
3. Past Medical History ....
   ....
   ....
4. Present Surgical History. ....
   ....
   ....
5. Past Surgical History. ....
   ....
   ....

6. Family History. ....
....
....

7. Personal History. ....
....
....

OBSTETRICAL HISTORY

S.No.	Year	Abortion	Prem	FT	Type of labour and mode of delivery	Gender	Live or Still Birth	Remark

LAB -INVESTIGATION

Hb	Blood Grouping	Blood Sugar	Urine		HIV	VDRL	Any Other
			Albumin	Sugar			

THE PUERPERIUM

Admitted to Postnatal Ward at AM/PM On:

POSTNATAL OBSERVATION CHART FOR MOTHER

Date	Day	Weight	Temp	Pulse	Resp	Fundal Height	Bowel	Urine	Lochia	Breast	Episiotomy Wound	Homen-sign

DELIVERY/OPERATION NOTES

Normal Vaginal Delivery

Type of labour : Spont /induced ....

Mode of delivery: Normal ....

Instrumental ....

Forcep/Vaccum..

Indication:..

Operation notes ....

....

....

....

....

....

....

CAESAREAN SECTION

Elective /Emergency..

Indication ....

Type: Lower Segment/Classical ....

Anaesthesia: Ga/Spinal/Epidural ....

Surgical Note..

1st Stage:..............................Hrs..Mins.

2nd Stage:............................Hrs..Mins.

3rd Stage:.............................Hrs..Mins.

Total : ....Hrs..Mins.

NEWBORN ASSESSMENT

Name of Baby...Gender.................................... Age...........

Apgar Score ....1min ....5 min Condition: Poor/Fair/Good

OBSERVATION CHART-BABY						
Date						
Day						
Weight						
Skin Colour						
Cord						
Eyes						
Mouth						
Urine						
Meconium						
Feeds						
Temperature						
Heart Rate						
Respiration						

Measurement:

Length ....cm

Head Circumference..cm

Chest Circumference...cm

Abdominal Circumference..cm

Reflexes:

Moro: ....

Sucking: ....

Swallowing: ....

Rooting:...

Grasping: ....

Vaccination: Age of the Baby...

BCG-Yes/No...

OPV-Yes/No...

Hep B-Yes/No ....

NURSING PROBLEMS AND RELATED OBJECTIVE OF CARE

Actual Nursing Problem for Mother and Baby

....

....

....

....

....

Potential Nursing Problems for Mother and Baby

....

....

....

....

NURSING CARE PLAN

ASSESSMENT	NSG DIAGNOSIS	GOAL	PLANNING	IMPLEMENTATION

Health Education to Mother

....

....

....

....

....

....

POSTNATAL AND NEONATAL CARE STUDY

IDENTIFICATION DATA

Name of Mother:..

W/o: ....

Age:..

Ward Name/Bed Number:..

Address: ....

Date of Admission:..

Date of Discharge:..

Obstetrical History – GPLA: ....

PAST MENSTRUAL HISTORY

LMP ....EDD ....Cycle..

HEALTH HISTORY

1. Past Obstetrical History..
....
....

2. Present Pregnancy History
   - I-trimester..
   ....
   ....
   - II-trimester..
   ....
   ....
   - III-trimester..
   ....
   ....

3. Past Medical History..
....
....

4. Present Surgical History. ....
....
....

5. Past Surgical History. ....
....
....

6. Family History. ....

....

....

7. Personal History. ....

....

....

OBSTETRICAL HISTORY

S.No.	Year	Abortion	Prem	FT	Type of labour and mode of delivery	Gender	Live or Still Birth	Remark

LAB -INVESTIGATION

Hb	Blood Grouping	Blood Sugar	Urine		HIV	VDRL	Any Other
			Albumin	Sugar			

THE PUERPERIUM

Admitted to Postnatal Ward at AM/PM On:

POSTNATAL OBSERVATION CHART FOR MOTHER

Date	Day	Weight	Temp	Pulse	Resp	Fundal Height	Bowel	Urine	Lochia	Breast	Episiotomy Wound	Homen-sign

DELIVERY/OPERATION NOTES

Normal Vaginal Delivery

Type of labour : Spont /induced ....

Mode of delivery: Normal ....

Instrumental ....

Forcep/Vaccum..

Indication:..

Operation notes ....

....

....

....

....

....

....

CAESAREAN SECTION

Elective /Emergency...

Indication ....

Type: Lower Segment/Classical ....

Anaesthesia: Ga/Spinal/Epidural ....

Surgical Note...

1st Stage:..............................Hrs...Mins.

2nd Stage:............................Hrs...Mins.

3rd Stage:.............................Hrs...Mins.

Total : ....Hrs...Mins.

NEWBORN ASSESSMENT

Name of Baby...Gender................................... Age...........

Apgar Score ....1min ....5 min Condition: Poor/Fair/Good

OBSERVATION CHART-BABY						
Date						
Day						
Weight						
Skin Colour						
Cord						
Eyes						
Mouth						
Urine						
Meconium						
Feeds						
Temperature						
Heart Rate						
Respiration						

Measurement:

Length ....cm

Head Circumference...cm

Chest Circumference...cm

Abdominal Circumference...cm

Reflexes:

Moro: ....

Sucking: ....

Swallowing: ....

Rooting:...

Grasping: ....

Vaccination: Age of the Baby...

BCG-Yes/No...

OPV-Yes/No...

Hep B-Yes/No ....

NURSING PROBLEMS AND RELATED OBJECTIVE OF CARE

Actual Nursing Problem for Mother and Baby

....

....

....

....

....

Potential Nursing Problems for Mother and Baby

....

....

....

....

NURSING CARE PLAN

ASSESSMENT	NSG DIAGNOSIS	GOAL	PLANNING	IMPLEMENTATION

Health Education to Mother

....

....

....

....

....

....

Clinical Care Record Book For Midwifery Program

(In accordance with INC Guidelines)

Priscilla John MSc (OBG)
Lecturer
Pal College of Nursing and Medical Sciences Haldwani
Nainital, Uttarakhand, India

Rekha Kumari MSc (OBG)
Lecturer
Pal College of Nursing and Medical Sciences Haldwani
Nainital, Uttarakhand, India

With Guidance of: **Dr Ratna Prakash** PhD PGDHE
Principal
Pal College of Nursing and Medical Sciences Haldwani
Nainital, Uttarakhand, India

Foreword
Ashok Pal

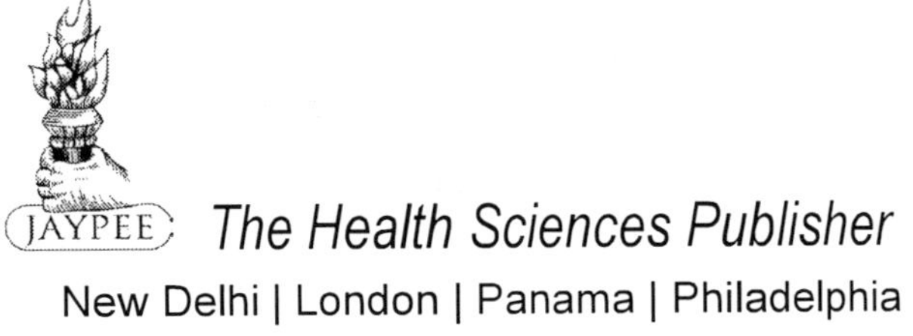

The Health Sciences Publisher
New Delhi | London | Panama | Philadelphia

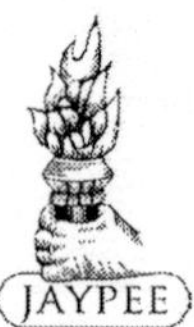

Jaypee Brothers Medical Publishers (P) Ltd

Headquarters

Jaypee Brothers Medical Publishers (P) Ltd
4838/24, Ansari Road, Daryaganj
New Delhi 110 002, India
Phone: +91-11-43574357
Fax: +91-11-43574314
Email: jaypee@jaypeebrothers.com

Overseas Offices

J.P. Medical Ltd
83, Victoria Street, London
SW1H 0HW (UK)
Phone: +44-20 3170 8910
Fax: +44-(0)20 3008 6180
Email: info@jpmedpub.com

Jaypee-Highlights Medical Publishers Inc
City of Knowledge, Bld. 237, Clayton
Panama City, Panama
Phone: +1 507-301-0496
Fax: +1 507-301-0499
Email: cservice@jphmedical.com

Jaypee Medical Inc
The Bourse
111, South Independence Mall East
Suite 835, Philadelphia, PA 19106, USA
Phone: +1 267-519-9789
Email: joe.rusko@jaypeebrothers.com

Jaypee Brothers Medical Publishers (P) Ltd
17/1-B, Babar Road, Block-B, Shaymali
Mohammadpur, Dhaka-1207
Bangladesh
Mobile: +08801912003485
Email: jaypeedhaka@gmail.com

Jaypee Brothers Medical Publishers (P) Ltd
Bhotahity, Kathmandu, Nepal
Phone: +977-9741283608
Email: Kathmandu@jaypeebrothers.com

Website: www.jaypeebrothers.com
Website: www.jaypeedigital.com

Clinical Care Record Book for Midwifery Program (In accordance with INC Guidelines)

First Edition: **2015, Reprint 2024**

ISBN : 978-93-5152-800-5

Printed in India

Foreword

Clinical Record Book is the compilation prepared for GNM and BSc Nursing Students. These students, on completion of the course, would support the health care delivery system at all health care arenas, where mother and child health is a major concern. GNM and BSc Nursing Professionals function as significant members of the Health Team at these levels. Hence, it is important to prepare the students of these courses suitably for performing their roles in the team.

The chapters are well thought of preliminaries to gently guide student's clinical learning experiences from 'known to unknown and simple to complex' phenomena that take place during birthing process. The language used is student friendly, materials are organized in logical sequence and learning experiences are designed to incorporate all the aspects of mother and child care from the conception to child birth and extending to new born care.

A well developed documentation system serves many purposes. Systematic documentation of learning experiences is an essential skill for all professional disciplines. The written documents are used as tools for evaluating student's learning. This compilation fulfils all these purposes, as aimed for.

It is a commendable task. I congratulate Mrs Priscilla John and Miss Rekha Kumari, teaching faculty of Pal College of Nursing and Medical Sciences for their thoughtful and organized efforts for facilitating student's learning.

Ashok Pal BE (Civil Engineering)
Director
Pal College of Nursing and Medical Sciences Haldwani
Nainital, Uttarakhand, India

Preface

This Clinical Record Book is prepared to accomplish the needs of all Midwifery students in their learning experiences. The content is arranged keeping in mind INC syllabus, requirements of GNM and BSc Nursing course and Indian Nursing Council standards.

This compilation aims to direct student's clinical reasoning in logical sequence with brief review of structural description of the body parts of mother and baby, participating in the process of birth. Thus, the initial chapters present brief review notes on the essential elements of birthing process, viz. female pelvis; fetal skull; fetal circulation and fetal lie. Following the chapters are organized incorporating the improvised steps of nursing process.

A brief description of the record book contents:

The logbook is designed to help undergraduate students to provide safe, sensitive and thoughtful care to their mother and child client unit.

The teaching and clinical supervision of teachers and efficient curriculum management enable the student to meet the unique requirement for practical and clinical aspects of midwifery.

Midwife is the person who assists women in childbirth. The students of this course must be capable and skillful in providing quality health care services.

Our main concern while compiling this clinical care record book is to consider the requirement of a midwifery students, their development of knowledge and skill in caring for each and every woman in pregnancy, labour and postpartum period. We hope that the minimum essential information added in this complication would benefit GNM and BSc nursing students as a record of their practical work.

I hope the content of this book will support the midwifery students in providing compassionate care to woman in pregnancy and newborn. I request all viewers and students to provide me with comments about each chapter, so that necessary changes could be done in next edition.

Dr Ratna Prakash

Acknowledgments

'We express our gratitude to Almighty God. For His grace and blessings, who has been the guiding force behind all our efforts'.

Our heartfelt thanks to Dr Ratna Prakash Professor, Principal of Pal College of Nursing and Medical Sciences for the encouragement, inspirations and support for taking up this project and guiding till its completion.

We express our Sincere Gratitude to Mr Ashok Pal, Director of the Institute for his constant encouragement in this work and for accepting to write the foreword for this book.

We are indebted to our colleagues for enriching this work by their expert suggestions and generally being there for us whenever we needed to fall back for their support.

We have put forth our sincere effort in compiling materials for *Clinical Care Record Book for Midwifery Program*, for the benefit of our students. We acknowledge and appreciate their indirect contribution in refining the materials as we got insights from their difficulty in using the formats.